Online Resources

Included with your purchase are multiple online resources. This includes the practice tests in an interactive format and a convenient study timer to help you manage your time.

Instructions for accessing these resources can be found on the last page of this book.

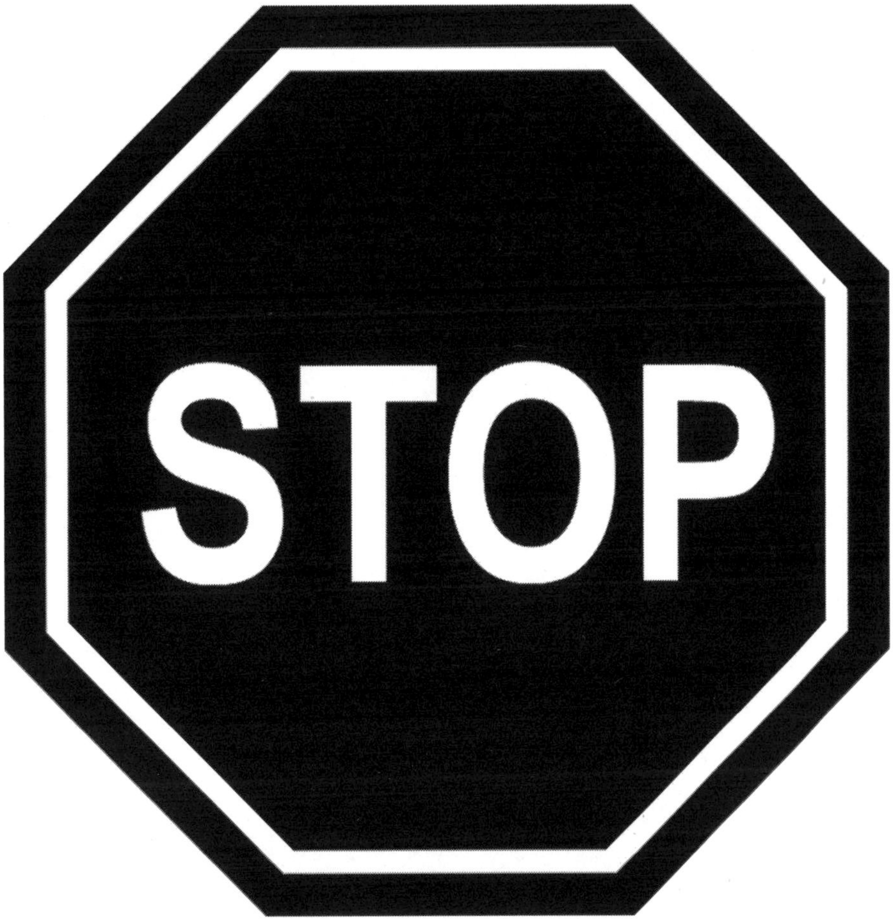

Kaplan® Nursing School Entrance Exam Prep

10 Practice Tests and Study Guide Book [Includes Audiobook]

Lydia Morrison

Written and edited by TPB Publishing.

ISBN 13: 9781637755372

Table of Contents

Welcome ---------- 1

Quick Overview ---------- 2

Test-Taking Strategies ---------- 3

Introduction for the Kaplan Nursing Entrance Exam ---------- 7

Study Prep Plan ---------- 9

Reading Comprehension ---------- 13

Practice Quiz ---------- 26

Answer Explanations ---------- 28

Writing ---------- 29

Practice Quiz ---------- 62

Answer Explanations ---------- 64

Mathematics ---------- 65

Practice Quiz ---------- 107

Answer Explanations ---------- 108

Science ---------- 109

Practice Quiz ---------- 143

Answer Explanations ---------- 144

Practice Test #1 ---------- 145

Answer Explanations #1 ---------- 163

Practice Test #2 ---------- 175

Answer Explanations #2 ---------- 196

Practice Test #3 ---------- 209

Answer Explanations #3 ---------- 229

Practice Tests #4 - #10 ---------- 242

Online Resources ---------- 245

Welcome

Dear Reader,

Welcome to your new Test Prep Books study guide! We are pleased that you chose us to help you prepare for your exam. There are many study options to choose from, and we appreciate you choosing us. Studying can be a daunting task, but we have designed a smart, effective study guide to help prepare you for what lies ahead.

Whether you're a parent helping your child learn and grow, a high school student working hard to get into your dream college, or a nursing student studying for a complex exam, we want to help give you the tools you need to succeed. We hope this study guide gives you the skills and the confidence to thrive, and we can't thank you enough for allowing us to be part of your journey.

In an effort to continue to improve our products, we welcome feedback from our customers. We look forward to hearing from you. Suggestions, success stories, and criticisms can all be communicated by emailing us at support@testprepbooks.com.

Sincerely,

Test Prep Books Team

Quick Overview

As you draw closer to taking your exam, effective preparation becomes more and more important. Thankfully, you have this study guide to help you get ready. Use this guide to help keep your studying on track and refer to it often.

This study guide contains several key sections that will help you be successful on your exam. The guide contains tips for what you should do the night before and the day of the test. Also included are test-taking tips. Knowing the right information is not always enough. Many well-prepared test takers struggle with exams. These tips will help equip you to accurately read, assess, and answer test questions.

A large part of the guide is devoted to showing you what content to expect on the exam and to helping you better understand that content. In this guide are practice test questions so that you can see how well you have grasped the content. Then, answer explanations are provided so that you can understand why you missed certain questions.

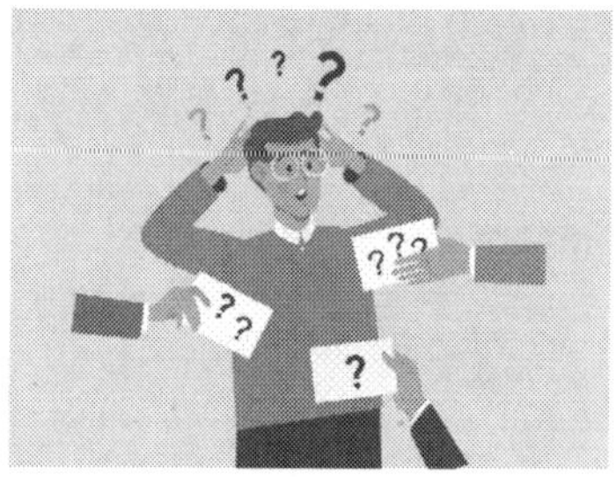

Don't try to cram the night before you take your exam. This is not a wise strategy for a few reasons. First, your retention of the information will be low. Your time would be better used by reviewing information you already know rather than trying to learn a lot of new information. Second, you will likely become stressed as you try to gain a large amount of knowledge in a short amount of time. Third, you will be depriving yourself of sleep. So be sure to go to bed at a reasonable time the night before. Being well-rested helps you focus and remain calm.

Be sure to eat a substantial breakfast the morning of the exam. If you are taking the exam in the afternoon, be sure to have a good lunch as well. Being hungry is distracting and can make it difficult to focus. You have hopefully spent lots of time preparing for the exam. Don't let an empty stomach get in the way of success!

When travelling to the testing center, leave earlier than needed. That way, you have a buffer in case you experience any delays. This will help you remain calm and will keep you from missing your appointment time at the testing center.

Be sure to pace yourself during the exam. Don't try to rush through the exam. There is no need to risk performing poorly on the exam just so you can leave the testing center early. Allow yourself to use all of the allotted time if needed.

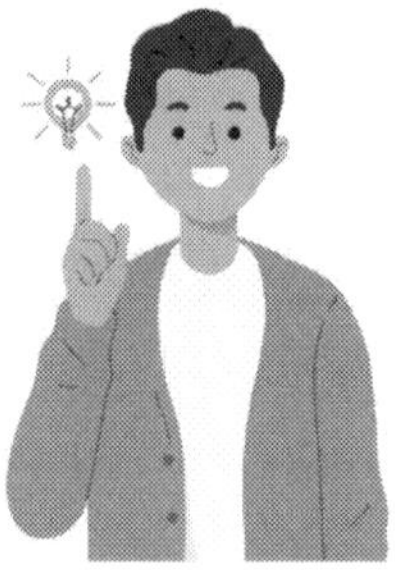

Remain positive while taking the exam even if you feel like you are performing poorly. Thinking about the content you should have mastered will not help you perform better on the exam.

Once the exam is complete, take some time to relax. Even if you feel that you need to take the exam again, you will be well served by some down time before you begin studying again. It's often easier to convince yourself to study if you know that it will come with a reward!

Test-Taking Strategies

1. Predicting the Answer

When you feel confident in your preparation for a multiple-choice test, try predicting the answer before reading the answer choices. This is especially useful on questions that test objective factual knowledge. By predicting the answer before reading the available choices, you eliminate the possibility that you will be distracted or led astray by an incorrect answer choice. You will feel more confident in your selection if you read the question, predict the answer, and then find your prediction among the answer choices. After using this strategy, be sure to still read all of the answer choices carefully and completely. If you feel unprepared, you should not attempt to predict the answers. This would be a waste of time and an opportunity for your mind to wander in the wrong direction.

2. Reading the Whole Question

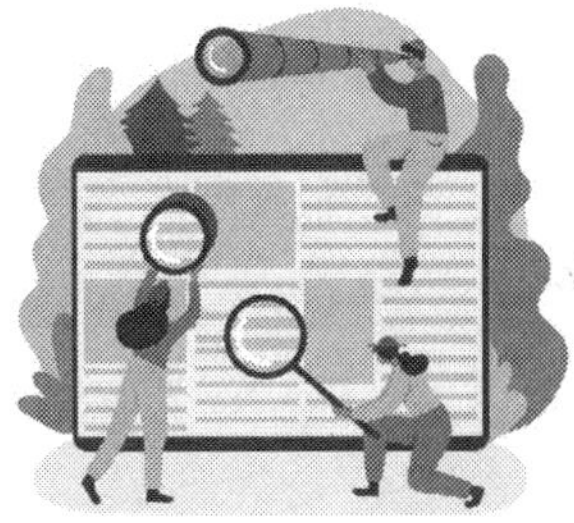

Too often, test takers scan a multiple-choice question, recognize a few familiar words, and immediately jump to the answer choices. Test authors are aware of this common impatience, and they will sometimes prey upon it. For instance, a test author might subtly turn the question into a negative, or he or she might redirect the focus of the question right at the end. The only way to avoid falling into these traps is to read the entirety of the question carefully before reading the answer choices.

3. Looking for Wrong Answers

Long and complicated multiple-choice questions can be intimidating. One way to simplify a difficult multiple-choice question is to eliminate all of the answer choices that are clearly wrong. In most sets of answers, there will be at least one selection that can be dismissed right away. If the test is administered on paper, the test taker could draw a line through it to indicate that it may be ignored; otherwise, the test taker will have to perform this operation mentally or on scratch paper. In either case, once the obviously incorrect answers have been eliminated, the remaining choices may be considered. Sometimes identifying the clearly wrong answers will give the test taker some information about the correct answer. For instance, if one of the remaining answer choices is a direct opposite of one of the eliminated answer choices, it may well be the correct answer. The opposite of obviously wrong is obviously right! Of course, this is not always the case. Some answers are obviously incorrect simply because they are irrelevant to the question being asked. Still, identifying and eliminating some incorrect answer choices is a good way to simplify a multiple-choice question.

4. Don't Overanalyze

Anxious test takers often overanalyze questions. When you are nervous, your brain will often run wild, causing you to make associations and discover clues that don't actually exist. If you feel that this may be a problem for you, do whatever you can to slow down during the test. Try taking a deep breath or counting to ten. As you read and consider the question, restrict yourself to the particular words used by the author. Avoid thought tangents about what the author *really* meant, or what he or she was *trying* to say. The only things that matter on a multiple-choice test are the words that are actually in the question. You must avoid reading too much into a multiple-choice question, or supposing that the writer meant something other than what he or she wrote.

5. No Need for Panic

It is wise to learn as many strategies as possible before taking a multiple-choice test, but it is likely that you will come across a few questions for which you simply don't know the answer. In this situation, avoid panicking. Because most multiple-choice tests include dozens of questions, the relative value of a single wrong answer is small. As much as possible, you should compartmentalize each question on a multiple-choice test. In other words, you should not allow your feelings about one question to affect your success on the others. When you find a question that you either don't understand or don't know how to answer, just take a deep breath and do your best. Read the entire question slowly and carefully. Try rephrasing the question a couple of different ways. Then, read all of the answer choices carefully. After eliminating obviously wrong answers, make a selection and move on to the next question.

6. Confusing Answer Choices

When working on a difficult multiple-choice question, there may be a tendency to focus on the answer choices that are the easiest to understand. Many people, whether consciously or not, gravitate to the answer choices that require the least concentration, knowledge, and memory. This is a mistake. When you come across an answer choice that is confusing, you should give it extra attention. A question might be confusing because you do not know the subject matter to which it refers. If this is the case, don't eliminate the answer before you have affirmatively settled on another. When you come across an answer choice of this type, set it aside as you look at the remaining choices. If you can confidently assert that one of the other choices is correct, you can leave the confusing answer aside. Otherwise, you will need to take a moment to try to better understand the confusing answer choice. Rephrasing is one way to tease out the sense of a confusing answer choice.

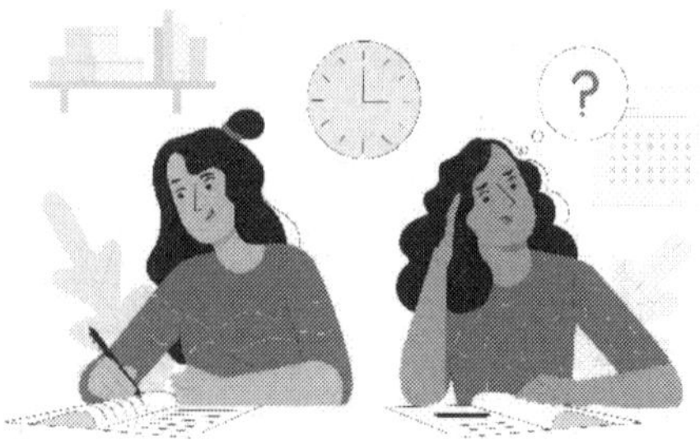

7. Your First Instinct

Many people struggle with multiple-choice tests because they overthink the questions. If you have studied sufficiently for the test, you should be prepared to trust your first instinct once you have carefully and completely read the question and all of the answer choices. There is a great deal of research suggesting that the mind can come to the correct conclusion very quickly once it has obtained all of the relevant information. At times, it may seem to you as if your intuition is working faster even than your reasoning mind. This may in fact be true. The knowledge you obtain while studying may be retrieved from your subconscious before you have a chance to work out the associations that support it. Verify your instinct by working out the reasons that it should be trusted.

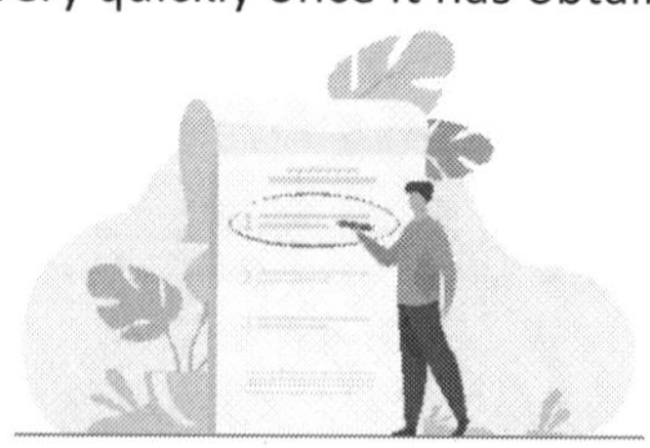

8. Key Words

Many test takers struggle with multiple-choice questions because they have poor reading comprehension skills. Quickly reading and understanding a multiple-choice question requires a mixture of skill and experience. To help with this, try jotting down a few key words and phrases on a piece of scrap paper. Doing this concentrates the process of reading and forces the mind to weigh the relative importance of the question's parts. In selecting words and phrases to write down, the test taker thinks about the question more deeply and carefully. This is especially true for multiple-choice questions that are preceded by a long prompt.

9. Subtle Negatives

One of the oldest tricks in the multiple-choice test writer's book is to subtly reverse the meaning of a question with a word like *not* or *except*. If you are not paying attention to each word in the question, you can easily be led astray by this trick. For instance, a common question format is, "Which of the following is...?" Obviously, if the question instead is, "Which of the following is not...?," then the answer will be quite different. Even worse, the test makers are aware of the potential for this mistake and will include one answer choice that would be correct if the question were not negated or reversed. A test taker who misses the reversal will find what he or she believes to be a correct answer and will be so confident that he or she will fail to reread the question and discover the original error. The only way to avoid this is to practice a wide variety of multiple-choice questions and to pay close attention to each and every word.

10. Reading Every Answer Choice

It may seem obvious, but you should always read every one of the answer choices! Too many test takers fall into the habit of scanning the question and assuming that they understand the question because they recognize a few key words. From there, they pick the first answer choice that answers the question they believe they have read. Test takers who read all of the answer choices might discover that one of the latter answer choices is actually *more* correct. Moreover, reading all of the answer choices can remind you of facts related to the question that can help you arrive at the correct answer. Sometimes, a misstatement or incorrect detail in one of the latter answer choices will trigger your memory of the subject and will enable you to find the right answer. Failing to read all of the answer choices is like not reading all of the items on a restaurant menu: you might miss out on the perfect choice.

11. Spot the Hedges

One of the keys to success on multiple-choice tests is paying close attention to every word. This is never truer than with words like *almost*, *most*, *some*, and *sometimes*. These words are called "hedges" because they indicate that a statement is not totally true or not true in every place and time. An absolute statement will contain no hedges, but in many subjects, the answers are not always straightforward or absolute. There are always exceptions to the rules in these subjects. For this reason, you should favor those multiple-choice questions that contain hedging language. The presence of

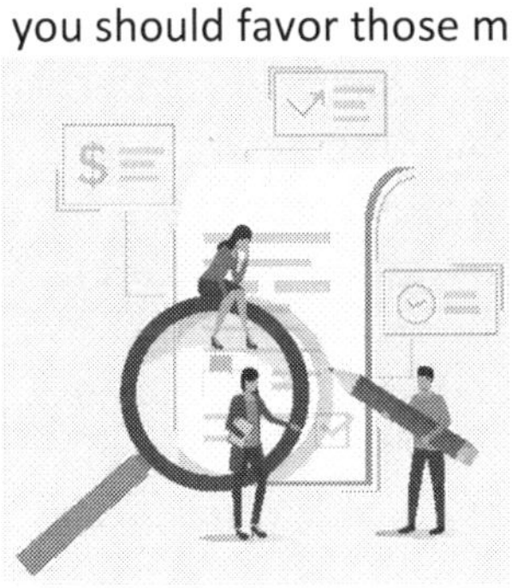

qualifying words indicates that the author is taking special care with his or her words, which is certainly important when composing the right answer. After all, there are many ways to be wrong, but there is only one way to be right! For this reason, it is wise to avoid answers that are absolute when taking a multiple-choice test. An absolute answer is one that says things are either all one way or all another. They often include words like *every*, *always*, *best*, and *never*. If you are taking a multiple-choice test in a subject that doesn't lend itself to absolute answers, be on your guard if you see any of these words.

12. Long Answers

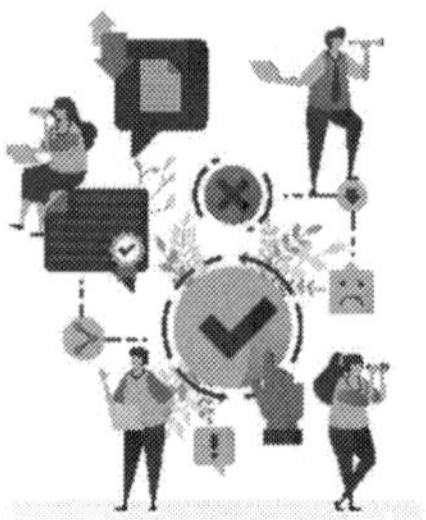

In many subject areas, the answers are not simple. As already mentioned, the right answer often requires hedges. Another common feature of the answers to a complex or subjective question are qualifying clauses, which are groups of words that subtly modify the meaning of the sentence. If the question or answer choice describes a rule to which there are exceptions or the subject matter is complicated, ambiguous, or confusing, the correct answer will require many words in order to be expressed clearly and accurately. In essence, you should not be deterred by answer choices that seem excessively long. Oftentimes, the author of the text will not be able to write the correct answer without offering some qualifications and modifications. Your job is to read the answer choices thoroughly and completely and to select the one that most accurately and precisely answers the question.

13. Restating to Understand

Sometimes, a question on a multiple-choice test is difficult not because of what it asks but because of how it is written. If this is the case, restate the question or answer choice in different words. This process serves a couple of important purposes. First, it forces you to concentrate on the core of the question. In order to rephrase the question accurately, you have to understand it well. Rephrasing the question will concentrate your mind on the key words and ideas. Second, it will present the information to your mind in a fresh way. This process may trigger your memory and render some useful scrap of information picked up while studying.

14. True Statements

Sometimes an answer choice will be true in itself, but it does not answer the question. This is one of the main reasons why it is essential to read the question carefully and completely before proceeding to the answer choices. Too often, test takers skip ahead to the answer choices and look for true statements. Having found one of these, they are content to select it without reference to the question above. The savvy test taker will always read the entire question before turning to the answer choices. Then, having settled on a correct answer choice, he or she will refer to the original question and ensure that the selected answer is relevant. The mistake of choosing a correct-but-irrelevant answer choice is especially common on questions related to specific pieces of objective knowledge.

15. No Patterns

One of the more dangerous ideas that circulates about multiple-choice tests is that the correct answers tend to fall into patterns. These erroneous ideas range from a belief that B and C are the most common right answers, to the idea that an unprepared test-taker should answer "A-B-A-C-A-D-A-B-A." It cannot be emphasized enough that pattern-seeking of this type is exactly the WRONG way to approach a multiple-choice test. To begin with, it is highly unlikely that the test maker will plot the correct answers according to some predetermined pattern. The questions are scrambled and delivered in a random order. Furthermore, even if the test maker was following a pattern in the assignation of correct answers, there is no reason why the test taker would know which pattern he or she was using. Any attempt to discern a pattern in the answer choices is a waste of time and a distraction from the real work of taking the test. A test taker would be much better served by extra preparation before the test than by reliance on a pattern in the answers.

Introduction for the Kaplan Nursing Entrance Exam

Function of the Test

The Kaplan Nursing School Admissions Test is designed to predict a nursing student's ability to be successful in one of any nursing schools in the United States. As such, it is a pre-admission assessment, and performance on the exam is considered as part of a nursing school candidate's application for program admissions. Kaplan believes that the test is a strong predictor of students' potential for success in their nursing education and pursuit of RN licensure. Most nursing programs across the country either require or recommend this pre-admissions assessment because they also believe that it aids in their admissions process, helping to identify strong candidates who are well-matched for their academic nursing program and future career as nurses.

The Kaplan Admissions Test assesses a candidate's knowledge and understanding of reading, math, the English language, and anatomy and physiology. It is a nationally-normed exam intended for students with a high school education. Nursing-specific education is not required to succeed on the test. General anatomy and physiology, similar to what should be learned in standard high school biology and science classes, is the only science on the exam. The rest assesses generalized knowledge in math, reading, and writing.

Test Administration

The Kaplan Nursing School Admissions Test is administered via computer. In general, candidates register for and take the exam at the nursing school where they are seeking admissions. Nursing programs offer the exam on a variety of dates during the academic year, particularly in the fall because scores are required as part of the application for admissions, which is typically due in the winter or early spring. Candidates should inquire about the specific dates and registration policies at the schools where they are seeking enrollment.

Test takers must bring a photo ID with them to the testing location. Retakes are permitted, but individual nursing programs are able to set their own policies on accepting retakes and the number of retakes allowable. Candidates desiring a retake should consult the programs they are interested in to verify their policies.

Test Format

The Kaplan Nursing School Admissions Test consist of 91 multiple-choice questions spread out over four sections. Test takers have 3 hours to take the test including breaks, and the actual testing time is 165 minutes. In the Reading section, test takers read various passages that may be about any topic such as science, the arts, and history. After each passage, test takers will answer a handful of questions that assess reading comprehension. There are 22 questions, which must be completed in 45 minutes. The math section also lasts 45 minutes, but it contains 28 questions that predominately focus on operations, conversions, ratios, and word problems. The Writing section, which is also 45 minutes, contains 21 questions that assess the candidate's command of the standard conventions of English language grammar, syntax, and writing mechanics. Test takers will identify grammatical, structural, and logical errors in written passages of a variety of topics pulled from all academic disciplines. Finally, in the 30-minute science section, test takers will answer 20 questions pertaining mostly to the physiology of select body systems such as the cardiovascular, gastrointestinal, immune, renal, and hematological, respiratory, and sensory systems. Neurology, electrolytes, and homeostasis concepts are also assessed.

The following table provides details of the four sections that comprise the test.

Section	Number of Multiple-Choice Questions	Time Limit (min)
Reading	22	45
Math	28	45
Writing	21	45
Science	20	30
Total	**91**	**165**

Scoring

Each of the four sections of the exam are scored separately based on the number of correct responses, and then the overall score, called the composite score, consists of the average of the section scores. Test takers and admissions counselors can thus see how the performance varied over the sections and as a whole. Scores are available immediately upon submitting the exam.

There is no set passing score for the Kaplan Nursing School Admissions Test; rather, individual nursing programs can set their own passing scores. Most programs throughout the country require a minimum score of somewhere between 60–69, although certain schools and programs may require a higher or lower score. Note that some schools do not have a specific passing score, but they consider any score in combination with the rest of the application materials such as overall and pre-nursing courses GPA, recommendations, and the rigor of courses attempted.

Study Prep Plan

1 **Schedule** - Use one of our study schedules below or come up with one of your own.

2 **Relax** - Test anxiety can hurt even the best students. There are many ways to reduce stress. Find the one that works best for you.

3 **Execute** - Once you have a good plan in place, be sure to stick to it.

One Week Study Schedule

Day 1	Reading Comprehension
Day 2	Writing
Day 3	Mathematics
Day 4	Science
Day 5	Practice Tests #1 & #2
Day 6	Practice Tests #3 & #4
Day 7	Take Your Exam!

Two Week Study Schedule

Day 1	Reading Comprehension	Day 8	Science
Day 2	Writing	Day 9	Hematological System
Day 3	Parts of Speech	Day 10	Practice Test #1
Day 4	Punctuation	Day 11	Practice Test #2
Day 5	Mathematics	Day 12	Practice Test #3
Day 6	Fractions	Day 13	Practice Test #4
Day 7	Word Problems	Day 14	Take Your Exam!

One Month Study Schedule

Day 1	Reading Comprehension	Day 11	Fractions	Day 21	Practice Questions
Day 2	Identifying a Writer's Purpose...	Day 12	Percentages	Day 22	Practice Test #1
Day 3	Practice Questions	Day 13	Word Problems	Day 23	Answer Explanations #1
Day 4	Writing	Day 14	Solving Simple Algebraic Problems	Day 24	Practice Test #2
Day 5	Parts of Speech	Day 15	Practice Questions	Day 25	Answer Explanations #2
Day 6	Sentences	Day 16	Science	Day 26	Practice Test #3
Day 7	Punctuation	Day 17	Gastrointestinal System	Day 27	Answer Explanations #3
Day 8	Practice Questions	Day 18	Neurology	Day 28	Practice Test #4
Day 9	Mathematics	Day 19	Homeostasis	Day 29	Answer Explanations #4
Day 10	Positive and Negative Numbers	Day 20	Sensory System	Day 30	Take Your Exam!

Build your own prep plan by visiting the Online Resources page.

Instructions and a QR code can be found on the last page of this guide.

As you study for your test, we'd like to take the opportunity to remind you that you are capable of great things! With the right tools and dedication, you truly can do anything you set your mind to. The fact that you are holding this book right now shows how committed you are. In case no one has told you lately, you've got this! Our intention behind including this coloring page is to give you the chance to take some time to engage your creative side when you need a little brain-break from studying. As a company, we want to encourage people like you to achieve their dreams by providing good quality study materials for the tests and certifications that improve careers and change lives. As individuals, many of us have taken such tests in our careers, and we know how challenging this process can be. While we can't come alongside you and cheer you on personally, we can offer you the space to recall your purpose, reconnect with your passion, and refresh your brain through an artistic practice. We wish you every success, and happy studying!

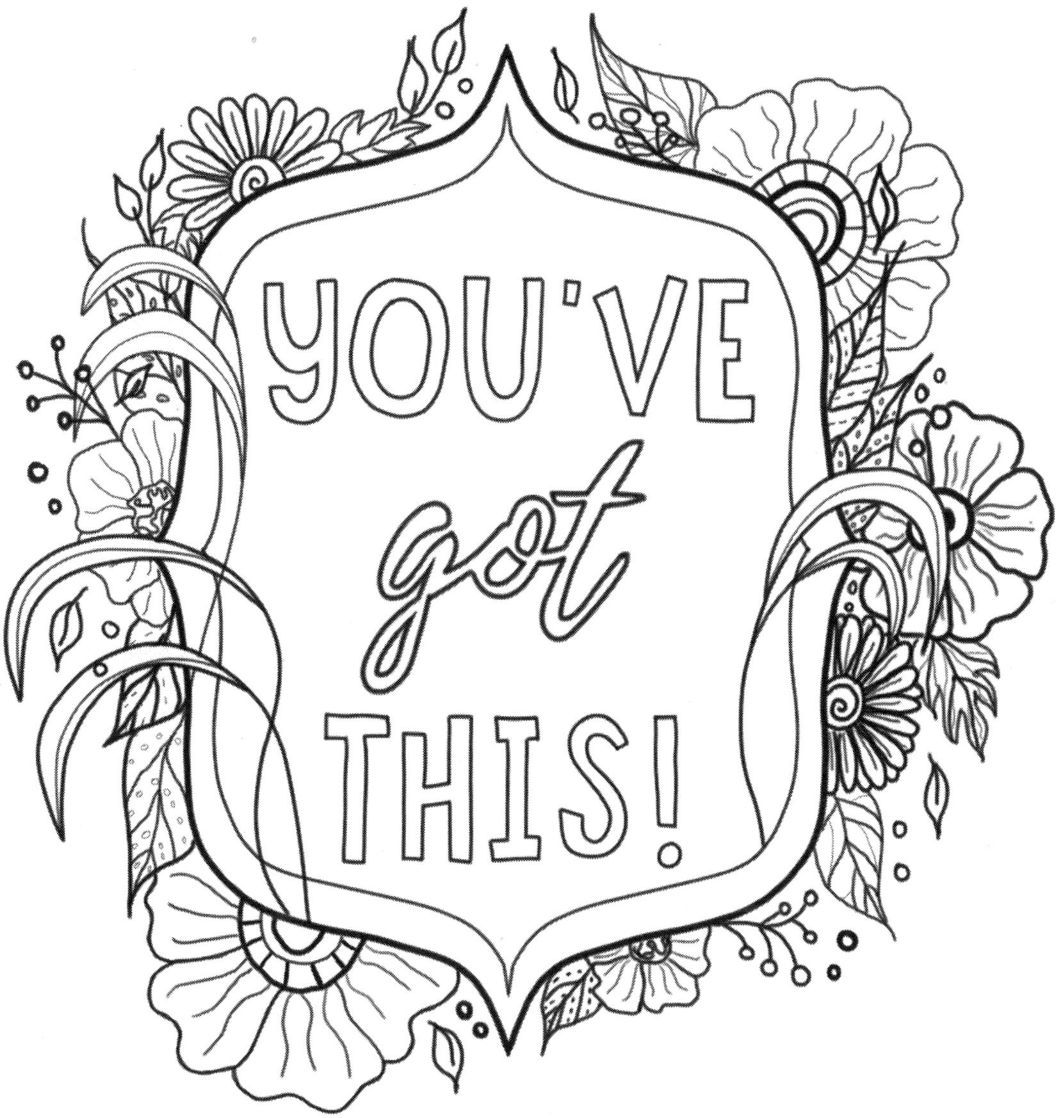

Reading Comprehension

Identifying the Main Idea

Topics and main ideas are critical parts of any writing. The **topic** is the subject matter of the piece, and it is a broader, more general term. The **main idea** is what the writer wants to say about that topic. The topic can be expressed in a word or two, but the main idea should be a complete thought.

The topic and main idea are usually easy to recognize in nonfiction writing. An author will likely identify the topic immediately in the first sentence of a passage or essay. The main idea is also typically presented in the introductory paragraph of an essay. In a single passage, the main idea may be identified in the first or the last sentence, but will likely be directly stated and easily recognized by the reader. Because it is not always stated immediately in a passage, it's important to carefully read the entire passage to identify the main idea.

Also remember that when most authors write, they want to make a point or send a message. This point or message of a text is known as the **theme**. Authors may state themes explicitly, like in *Aesop's Fables*. More often, especially in modern literature, readers must infer the theme based on text details. Usually after carefully reading and analyzing an entire text, the reader can identify the theme. Typically, the longer the piece, the more themes you will encounter, though often one theme dominates the rest, as evidenced by the author's purposeful revisiting of it throughout the passage.

The main idea should not be confused with the thesis statement. A **thesis statement** is a clear statement of the writer's specific stance, and can often be found in the introduction of a nonfiction piece. The main idea is more of an overview of the entire piece, while the thesis is a specific sentence found in that piece.

In order to illustrate the main idea, a writer will use **supporting details** in a passage. These details can provide evidence or examples to help make a point. Supporting details are most commonly found in nonfiction pieces that seek to inform or persuade the reader.

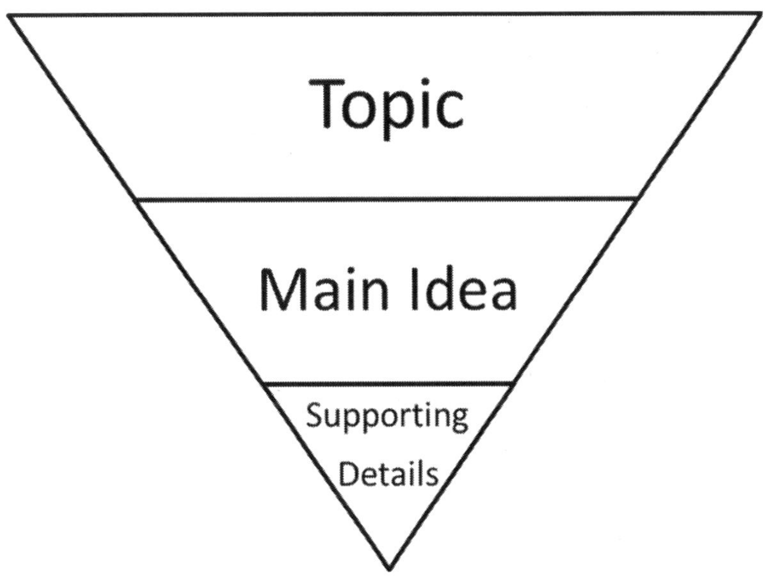

As a reader, you will want to carefully examine the author's supporting details to be sure they are credible. Consider whether they provide evidence of the author's point and whether they directly support the main idea. You might find that an author has used a shocking statistic to grab your attention, but that the statistic doesn't really support the main idea, so it isn't being effectively used in the piece.

Identifying Supporting Details

Supporting details help readers better develop and understand the main idea. Supporting details answer questions like *who, what, where, when, why,* and *how*. Different types of supporting details include examples, facts and statistics, anecdotes, and sensory details.

Persuasive and informative texts often use supporting details. In persuasive texts, authors attempt to make readers agree with their points of view, and supporting details are often used as "selling points." If authors make a statement, they need to support the statement with evidence in order to adequately persuade readers. Informative texts use supporting details such as examples and facts to inform readers. Review the"Cheetahs" passage to find examples of supporting details.

> Cheetahs are one of the fastest mammals on the land, reaching up to 70 miles an hour over short distances. Even though cheetahs can run as fast as 70 miles an hour, they usually only have to run half that speed to catch up with their choice of prey. Cheetahs cannot maintain a fast pace over long periods of time because their bodies will overheat. After a chase, cheetahs need to rest for approximately 30 minutes prior to eating or returning to any other activity.

In the example, supporting details include:

- Cheetahs reach up to 70 miles per hour over short distances.
- They usually only have to run half that speed to catch up with their prey.
- Cheetahs will overheat if they exert a high speed over longer distances.
- Cheetahs need to rest for 30 minutes after a chase.

Look at the diagram below (applying the cheetah example) to help determine the hierarchy of topic, main idea, and supporting details.

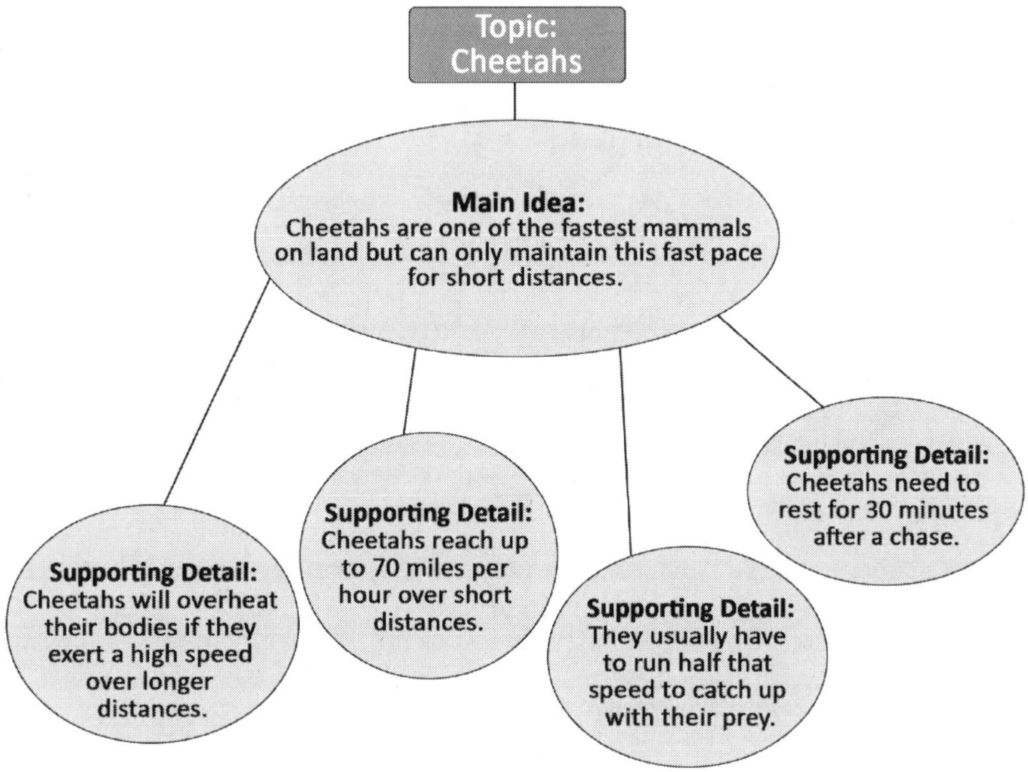

Finding the Meaning of Words and Phrases in Context

There will be many occasions in one's reading career in which an unknown word or a word with multiple meanings will pop up. There are ways of determining what these words or phrases mean that do not require the use of the dictionary, which is especially helpful during a test where one may not be available. Even outside of the exam, knowing how to derive an understanding of a word via **context clues** will be a critical skill in the real world. The context is the circumstances in which a story or a passage is happening, and can usually be found in the series of words directly before or directly after the word or phrase in question. The clues are the words that hint towards the meaning of the unknown word or phrase. The author may use synonyms or antonyms that you can use. **Synonyms** refer to words that have the same meaning as another word (e.g., instructor/teacher/educator, canine/dog, feline/cat, herbivore/vegetarian). **Antonyms** refer to words that have the opposite meaning as another word (e.g., true/false, up/down, in/out, right/wrong).

There may be questions that ask about the meaning of a particular word or phrase within a passage. There are a couple ways to approach these kinds of questions:

- Define the word or phrase in a way that is easy to comprehend (using context clues).
- Try out each answer choice in place of the word.

To demonstrate, here's an example from *Alice in Wonderland*:

> Alice was beginning to get very tired of sitting by her sister on the bank, and of having nothing to do: once or twice she peeped into the book her sister was reading, but it had no pictures or conversations in it, "and what is the use of a book," thought Alice, "without pictures or conversations?"

Q: As it is used in the selection, the word peeped means:

Using the first technique, before looking at the answers, define the word *peeped* using context clues and then find the matching answer. Then, analyze the entire passage in order to determine the meaning, not just the surrounding words.

To begin, imagine a blank where the word should be and put a synonym or definition there: "once or twice she ___ into the book her sister was reading." The context clue here is the book. It may be tempting to put *read* where the blank is, but notice the preposition word *into*. One does not read into a book, one simply reads a book, and since reading a book requires that it is seen with a pair of eyes, then *look* would make the most sense to put into the blank: "once or twice she looked into the book her sister was reading."

Once an easy-to-understand word or synonym has been supplanted, check to make sure it makes sense with the rest of the passage. What happened after she looked into the book? She thought to herself how a book without pictures or conversations is useless. This situation in its entirety makes sense.

Now check the answer choices for a match:

a. To make a high-pitched cry
b. To smack
c. To look curiously
d. To pout

Since the word was already defined, answer choice (c) is the best option.

Using the second technique, replace the figurative blank with each of the answer choices and determine which one is the most appropriate. Remember to look further into the passage to clarify that they work, because they could still make sense out of context.

> Once or twice she made a high-pitched cry into the book her sister was reading.
>
> Once or twice she smacked the book her sister was reading.
>
> Once or twice she looked curiously into the book her sister was reading.
>
> Once or twice she pouted into the book her sister was reading.

For Choice *A,* it does not make much sense in any context for a person to cry into a book, unless maybe something terrible has happened in the story. Given that afterward Alice thinks to herself how useless a book without pictures is, this option does not make sense within context.

For Choice *B,* smacking a book someone is reading may make sense if the rest of the passage indicates there a reason for doing so. If Alice was angry or her sister had shoved it in her face, then maybe smacking the book would make sense within context. However, since whatever she does with the book causes her to think, "what is the use of a book without pictures or conversations?" then answer Choice *B* is not an appropriate answer.

Answer Choice *C* fits well within context, given her subsequent thoughts on the matter.

Answer Choice *D* does not make sense in context or grammatically, as people do not pout into things.

This is a simple example to illustrate the techniques outlined above. There may, however, be a question in which all of the definitions are correct and also make sense out of context, in which the appropriate context clues will really need to be observed in order to determine the correct answer. For example, here is another passage from *Alice in Wonderland*:

> ... but when the Rabbit actually took a watch out of its waistcoat pocket, and looked at it, and then hurried on, Alice <u>started</u> to her feet, for it flashed across her mind that she had never before seen a rabbit with either a waistcoat-pocket or a watch to take out of it, and burning with curiosity, she ran across the field after it, and was just in time to see it pop down a large rabbit-hole under the hedge.

Q: As it is used in the passage, the word <u>started</u> means _____.
- a. to turn on
- b. to begin
- c. to move quickly
- d. to be surprised

All of these words qualify as a definition of start, but using context clues, the correct answer can be identified using one of the two techniques above. It's easy to see that one does not turn on, begin, or be surprised to one's feet. The selection also states that she "ran across the field after it," indicating that she was in a hurry. Therefore, to move quickly would make the most sense in this context.

The same strategies can be applied to vocabulary that may be completely unfamiliar. In this case, focus on the words before or after the unknown word in order to determine its definition. Take this sentence, for example:

> Sam was such a <u>miser</u> that he forced Andrew to pay him twelve cents for the candy, even though he had a large inheritance and he knew his friend was poor.

For vocabulary questions, it may be necessary to apply some critical thinking skills when something isn't explicitly stated within the passage. Think about the implications of the passage, or what the text is trying to say. With this example, it is important to realize that it is considered unusually stingy for a person to demand so little money from someone instead of just letting their friend have the candy, especially if this person is already wealthy. Hence, a <u>miser</u> is a greedy or stingy individual.

Another useful strategy in determining the meaning of an unknown word is to look at the word's prefix and suffix.

A **prefix** is a word, letter, or number that is placed before another. It adjusts or qualifies the original word's meaning.

Four prefixes represent 97% of English words with prefixes. They are:

- *dis-* means "not" or "opposite of"; *dis*abled
- in-, im-, il-, ir- mean "not"; illiterate
- *re-* means "again"; *re*turn
- *un-* means "not"; *un*predictable

Other commons prefixes include:

- *anti-* means "against"; antibacterial
- *fore-* means "before"; forefront
- *mis-* means "wrongly"; misunderstand
- *non-* means "not"; nonsense
- *over-* means "over"; overabundance
- *pre-* means "before"; preheat
- *super-* means "above"; superman

The official definition of a **suffix** is "a morpheme added at the end of a word to form a derivative." In simpler terms, that means a suffix is a letter or group of letters added at the end of a word to form another word. The word created with the addition is either a different tense of the same word (*help + ed = helped)* or a new word (*help + ful = helpful).*

They are:

- *-ed* is used to make present tense verbs into past tense verbs; wash*ed*
- *-ing* is used to make a present tense verb into a present participle verb; wash*ing*
- *-ly* is used to make characteristic of; love*ly*
- *-s* or *–es* are used to make more than one; chair*s* or box*es*

Other common suffixes include:

- *-able* means can be done; deplor*able*
- *-al* means having characteristics of; comic*al*
- *-est* means comparative; great*est*
- *-ful* means full of; wonder*ful*
- *-ism* means belief in; commun*ism*
- *-less* means without; faith*less*
- *-ment* means action or process; accomplish*ment*
- *-ness* means state of; happi*ness*
- *-ize* means to render, to make; terror*ize,* steril*ize*
- *-ise* means ditto, only this is primarily the British variant of *–ize;* surpr*ise,* advert*ise*
- -ced means go; spelling variations include -cede (concede, recede); -ceed (only three: proceed, exceed, succeed); -sede (the only one: supersede)

(Note: In some of the examples above, the *e* has been deleted.)

Questions about complex vocabulary may not be explicitly asked, but this is a useful skill to know. If there is an unfamiliar word while reading a passage and its definition goes unknown, it is possible to miss out on a critical message that could inhibit the ability to appropriately answer the questions.

Practicing this technique in daily life will sharpen this ability to derive meanings from context clues with ease.

Identifying a Writer's Purpose and Tone

Purpose

Writing can be classified under four passage types: narrative, expository, technical, and persuasive. Though these types are not mutually exclusive, one form tends to dominate the rest. By recognizing the *type* of passage you're reading, you gain insight into *how* you should read. If you're reading a narrative, you can assume the author intends to entertain, which means you may skim the text without losing meaning. A technical document might require a close read because skimming the passage might cause the reader to miss salient details.

1. **Narrative writing**, at its core, is the art of storytelling. For a narrative to exist, certain elements must be present. It must have characters. While many characters are human, characters could be defined as anything that thinks, acts, and talks like a human. For example, many recent movies, such as *Lord of the Rings* and *The Chronicles of Narnia*, include animals, fantastical creatures, and even trees that behave like humans. It must have a plot or sequence of events. Typically, those events follow a standard plot diagram, but recent trends start *in medias res* or in the middle (near the climax). In this instance, foreshadowing and flashbacks often fill in plot details. Along with characters and a plot, there must also be conflict. Conflict is usually divided into two types: internal and external. Internal conflict indicates the character is in turmoil. Internal conflicts are presented through the character's thoughts. External conflicts are visible. Types of external conflict include a person versus nature, another person, and society.

2. **Expository writing** is detached and to the point. Since expository writing is designed to instruct or inform, it usually involves directions and steps written in second person ("you" voice) and lacks any persuasive or narrative elements. Sequence words such as *first*, *second*, and *third*, or *in the first place*, *secondly*, and *lastly* are often given to add fluency and cohesion. Common examples of expository writing include instructor's lessons, cookbook recipes, and repair manuals.

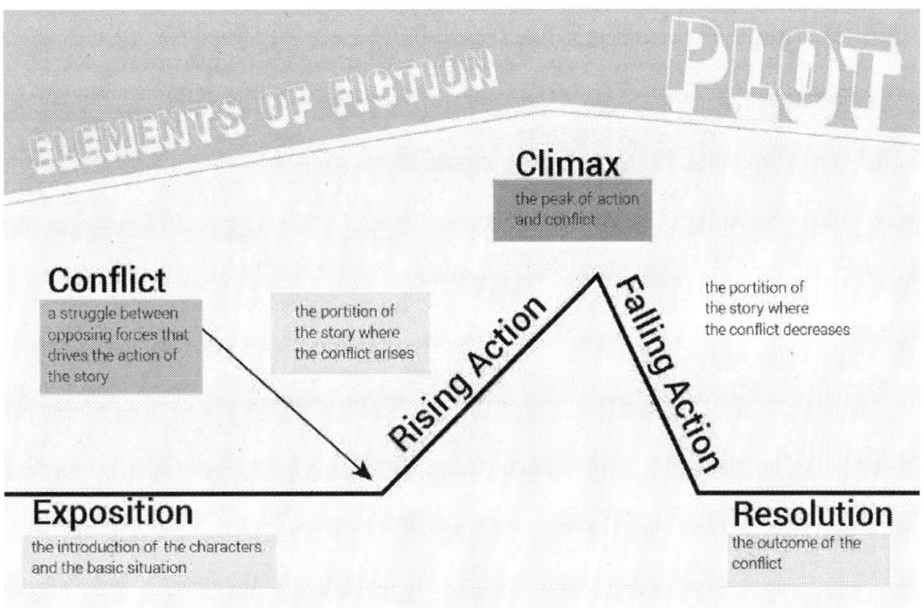

3. Due to its empirical nature, **descriptive writing** is filled with steps, charts, graphs, data, and statistics. The goal of technical writing is to advance understanding in a field through the scientific method. Experts such as teachers, doctors, or mechanics use words unique to the profession in which they operate. These words, which often incorporate acronyms, are called **jargon**. Technical writing is a type of expository writing but is not meant to be understood by the general public. Instead, technical writers assume readers have received a formal education in a particular field of study and need no explanation as to what the jargon means. Imagine a doctor trying to understand a diagnostic reading for a car or a mechanic trying to interpret lab results. Only professionals with proper training will fully comprehend the text.

4. **Persuasive writing** is designed to change opinions and attitudes. The topic, stance, and arguments are found in the thesis, positioned near the end of the introduction. Later supporting paragraphs offer relevant quotations, paraphrases, and summaries from primary or secondary sources, which are then interpreted, analyzed, and evaluated. The goal of persuasive writers is not to stack quotes but to develop original ideas by using sources as a starting point. Good persuasive writing makes powerful arguments with valid sources and thoughtful analysis. Poor persuasive writing is riddled with bias and logical fallacies. Sometimes, logical and illogical arguments are sandwiched together in the same piece. Therefore, readers should display skepticism when reading persuasive arguments.

Readers should always identify the author's position or stance in a text. No matter how objective a piece may seem, assume the author has preconceived beliefs. Reduce the likelihood of accepting an invalid argument by looking for multiple articles on the topic, including those with varying opinions. If several opinions point in the same direction, and are backed by reputable peer-reviewed sources, it's more likely the author has a valid argument. Positions that run contrary to widely held beliefs and existing data should invite scrutiny. There are exceptions to the rule, so be a careful consumer of information.

Tone

Tone refers to the writer's attitude toward the subject matter. Tone conveys how the writer feels about characters, situations, events, ideas, etc.

A lot of nonfiction writing has a neutral tone, which is an important one for the writer to use. A **neutral tone** demonstrates that the writer is presenting a topic impartially and letting the information speak for itself. On the other hand, nonfiction writing can be just as effective and appropriate if the tone isn't neutral. The following short passage provides an example of tone in nonfiction writing:

> Seat belts save more lives than any other automobile safety feature. Many studies show that airbags save lives as well; however, not all cars have airbags. For instance, some older cars don't. Furthermore, air bags aren't entirely reliable. For example, studies show that in 15% of accidents airbags don't deploy as designed, but, on the other hand, seat belt malfunctions are extremely rare. The number of highway fatalities has plummeted since laws requiring seat belt usage were enacted.

In this passage, the writer mostly chooses to retain a neutral tone when presenting information. If instead, the author chose to include their own personal experience of losing a friend or family member in a car accident, the tone would change dramatically. Or, if the author used words and phrases such as, "Ever since the government required individuals to wear seat belts, the amount of hard-working American lives that have been saved is extraordinary! Such a small task to undertake has changed the entire country." The tone would no longer be neutral and would show the reader the seriousness, joy, sadness, etc. of the situation. The tone would no longer be neutral and would show that the writer has a personal stake in the content, allowing him or her to interpret the information in a different way. When analyzing tone, the reader should consider what the writer is trying to achieve in the text and how they *create* the tone using style.

The following two poems and the essay concern the theme of death and are presented to demonstrate how to evaluate tone:

Poem 1

How wonderful is Death,

Death, and his brother Sleep!

One, pale as yonder waning moon

With lips of lurid blue;

The other, rosy as the morn

When throned on ocean's wave

It blushes o'er the world;

Yet both so passing wonderful!

"Queen Mab," Percy Bysshe Shelley

Poem 2

After great pain, a formal feeling comes –

The Nerves sit ceremonious, like Tombs –

The stiff Heart questions 'was it He, that bore,'

And 'Yesterday, or Centuries before'?

The Feet, mechanical, go round –

A Wooden way

Of Ground, or Air, or Ought –

Regardless grown,

A Quartz contentment, like a stone –

This is the Hour of Lead –

Remembered, if outlived,

As Freezing persons, recollect the Snow –

First – Chill – then Stupor – then the letting go –

"After Great Pain, A Formal Feeling Comes," Emily Dickinson

Essay 1

The Process of Dying

> Death occurs in several stages. The first stage is the pre-active stage, which occurs a few days to weeks before death, in which the desire to eat and drink decreases, and the person may feel restless, irritable, and anxious. The second stage is the active stage, where the skin begins to cool, breathing becomes difficult as the lungs become congested (known as the "death rattle"), and the person loses control of their bodily fluids.
>
> Once death occurs, there are also two stages. The first is clinical death, when the heart stops pumping blood and breathing ceases. This stage lasts approximately 4-6 minutes, and during this time, it is possible for a victim to be resuscitated via CPR or a defibrillator. After 6 minutes however, the oxygen stores within the brain begin to deplete, and the victim enters biological death. This is the point of no return, as the cells of the brain and vital organs begin to die, a process that is irreversible.

Readers should notice the differences in the word choices between the two poems. Percy Shelley's word choices— "wonderful," "rosy," "blushes," "ocean"—surrounding death indicates that he views death in a welcoming manner as his words carry positive charges. However, Dickinson's word choices— "pain," "wooden," "stone," "lead," "chill," "tombs"—carry negative connotations, which indicates an aversion to death. **Connotation** refers to the implied meaning of a word or phrase. Connotations are the ideas or feelings that words or phrase invoke other than their literal meaning. In contrast, the expository passage has no emotionally-charged words of any kind, and seems to view death simply as a process that happens, neither welcoming nor fearing it. The tone in this passage is neutral.

Distinguishing Between Fact and Opinion

It is important to distinguish between fact and opinion when reading a piece of writing. Readers should check the validity and accuracy of the facts that an author presents. When authors use opinion, they are sharing their own thoughts and feelings about the subject. You can recognize a piece that relies on opinion when the author uses words like *think, feel, believe,* or *in my opinion,* though these words won't always appear in an opinion piece, especially if it is formally written. An author's opinion may be backed up by facts, which gives it more credibility, but it should not be taken as fact. A critical reader should be wary of an author's opinion, especially if it is only supported by other opinions.
Here are some examples of facts versus opinions:

Facts	**Opinions**
There are 9 innings in a game of baseball.	Baseball games run too long.
Eisenhower expanded Social Security.	This action was helpful for the country.
McDonalds has stores in 118 countries.	McDonalds has the best hamburgers.

As a critical reader, you must examine the facts that are used to support the author's argument. You can check the facts against other sources to be sure they are correct. You can also check the validity of the sources used to be sure they are credible, academic, and peer reviewed sources. Consider that when an author uses another person's opinion to support the argument, even if it is an expert's opinion, it is still only an opinion, and should not be taken as fact. A strong argument uses valid, measurable facts to support ideas. Even then, the reader may disagree with the argument, as it is rooted in the author's **assumptions**, which are the author's personal beliefs.

Making Logical Inferences

Critical readers should be able to make inferences. Making an **inference** requires the reader to read between the lines and look for what is implied rather than what is explicitly stated. That means, using information that is known from the text, the reader is able to make a logical assumption about information that is not explicitly stated but is probably true. Read the following passage:

> "Hey, do you want to meet my new puppy?" Jonathan asked.
>
> "Oh, I'm sorry but please don't—" Jacinta began to protest, but before she could finish Jonathan had already opened the passenger side door of his car and a perfect white ball of fur came bouncing towards Jacinta.
>
> "Isn't he the cutest?" beamed Jonathan.
>
> "Yes—achoo! —he's pretty—aaaachooo!!—adora—aaa—aaaachoo!" Jacinta managed to say in between sneezes. "But if you don't mind, I—I—achoo! —need to go inside."

Which of the following can be inferred from Jacinta's reaction to the puppy?

a. She hates animals.
b. She is allergic to dogs.
c. She prefers cats to dogs.
d. She is angry at Jonathan.

An inference requires the reader to consider the information presented and then form their own idea about what is probably true. Based on the details in the passage, what is the best answer to the question? Important details to pay attention to in the passage include the tone of Jacinta's dialogue, as well as her reaction itself, which is a long string of sneezes. Choices *A* and *D* both express strong emotions ("hates" and "angry") that are not evident in Jacinta's speech or actions. Choice *C* mentions cats, but there is nothing in the passage to indicate Jacinta's feelings about cats. Choice *B*, "she is allergic to dogs," is the most logical choice. Based on the fact she began sneezing as soon as a fluffy dog approached her, it makes sense to guess that Jacinta might be allergic to dogs. Using the clues in the passage, it is reasonable to guess that this is true even though Jacinta never directly states, "Sorry, I'm allergic to dogs!"

Making inferences is crucial because literary texts often avoid presenting complete and direct information to readers about characters' thoughts or feelings, or they present the information in an unclear way, leaving it up to the reader to interpret clues given in the text. In order to make inferences while reading, readers should ask themselves:

- What details are being presented in the text?
- Is there any important information that seems to be missing?
- Based on the information that the author *does* include, what else is probably true?
- Is this inference reasonable based on what is already known?

Conclusions

Active readers should also draw conclusions. When doing so, the reader should ask the following questions: What is this piece about? What does the author believe? Does this piece have merit? Do I believe the author? Would this piece support my argument? The reader should first determine the author's intent. Identify the author's viewpoint and connect relevant evidence to support it. Readers may then move to the most important step: deciding whether to agree and determining whether they are correct. Always read cautiously and critically. Interact with text, and record reactions in the margins. These active reading skills help determine not only what the author thinks, but what you think as the reader.

Evaluating an Argument and its Specific Claims

It's important to evaluate the author's supporting details to be sure that the details are credible, provide evidence of the author's point, and directly support the main idea. Though shocking statistics grab readers' attention, their use could be ineffective information in the text. Details like this are crucial to understanding the passage and evaluating how well the author presents their argument and evidence.

Readers **draw conclusions** about what an author has presented. This helps them better understand what the writer has intended to communicate and whether or not they agree with what the author has offered. There are a few ways to determine a logical conclusion, but careful reading is the most important. It's helpful to read a passage a few times, noting details that seem important to the text. Sometimes, readers arrive at a conclusion that is different than what the writer intended or come up with more than one conclusion.

Evidence

It is important to distinguish between **fact and opinion** when reading a text. When an author presents facts, such as statistics or data, readers should be able to check those facts and make sure they are accurate. When authors use opinion, they are sharing their own thoughts and feelings about a subject.

Textual evidence helps readers draw a conclusion about a passage. **Textual evidence** refers to information—facts and examples that support the main point; it will likely come from outside sources and can be in the form of quoted or paraphrased material. In order to draw a conclusion from evidence, it's important to examine the credibility and validity of that evidence as well as how (and if) it relates to the main idea.

Credibility

Critical readers examine the facts used to support an author's argument. They check the facts against other sources to be sure those facts are correct. They also check the validity of the sources used to be sure those sources are credible, academic, and/or peer reviewed. Consider that when an author uses another person's opinion to support their argument, even if it is an expert's opinion, it is still only an opinion and should not be taken as fact. A strong argument uses valid, measurable facts to support ideas. Even then, the reader may disagree with the argument as it may be rooted in their personal beliefs.

An authoritative argument may use the facts to sway the reader. Because of this, a writer may choose to only use the information and expert opinion that supports their viewpoint.

Appeal to Emotion

An author's argument might also appeal to readers' emotions, perhaps by including personal stories and **anecdotes** (a short narrative of a specific event).

The next example presents an appeal to emotion. By sharing the personal anecdote of one student and speaking about emotional topics like family relationships, the author invokes the reader's empathy in asking them to reconsider the school rule.

> Our school should abolish its current ban on campus cell phone use. If students aren't able to use their phones during the school day, many of them feel isolated from their loved ones. For example, last semester, one student's grandmother had a heart attack in the morning. However, because he couldn't use his cell phone, the student didn't know about his grandmother's accident until the end of the day—when she had already passed away, and it was too late to say goodbye. By preventing students from contacting their friends and family, our school is placing undue stress and anxiety on students.

Counterarguments

If an author presents a differing opinion or a **counterargument** in order to refute it, the reader should consider how and why the information is being presented. It is meant to strengthen the original argument and shouldn't be confused with the author's intended conclusion, but it should also be considered in the reader's final evaluation. On the contrary, sometimes authors will concede to an opposing argument by recognizing the validity the other side has to offer. A concession will allow readers to see both sides of the argument in an unbiased light, thereby increasing the credibility of the author.

Authors can also reflect **bias** if they ignore an opposing viewpoint or present their side in an unbalanced way. A strong argument considers the opposition and finds a way to refute it. Critical readers should look for an unfair or one-sided presentation of the argument and be skeptical, as a bias may be present. Even if this bias is unintentional, if it exists in the writing, the reader should be wary of the validity of the argument.

Summarizing

A **summary** is a shortened version of the original text, written by the reader in their own words. In order to effectively summarize a more complex text, it is necessary to fully understand the original source, and to highlight the major points covered. It may be helpful to outline the original text to get a big picture view of it, and to avoid getting bogged down in the minor details. For example, a summary wouldn't need to include a specific statistic from the original source unless it was the major focus of the text. Also, it's important for readers to use their own words, but to retain the original meaning of the passage. The key to a good summary is to emphasize the main idea without changing the focus of the original information.

Paraphrasing calls for the reader to take a small part of the passage and list or describe its main points. Paraphrasing is more than rewording the original passage, though. As with summary, a paraphrase should be written in the reader's own words, while still retaining the meaning of the original source. The main difference between summarizing and paraphrasing is the length of the original passage. A summary would be appropriate for a much larger piece, while paraphrase might focus on just a few lines of text. Effective paraphrasing will indicate an understanding of the original source, yet still help the reader expand on their interpretation. A paraphrase should neither add new information nor remove essential facts that will change the meaning of the source.

Practice Quiz

The next five questions are based on the following passage:

Christopher Columbus is often credited with discovering America. This is a matter of perspective; America was unknown to fifteenth-century Europe, but bear in mind that the places he "discovered" were already filled with people who had been living there for centuries. What's more, Christopher Columbus was not the first European explorer to reach the Americas! Rather, it was Leif Erikson who first came to the New World and contacted the natives nearly 500 years before Christopher Columbus.

Leif Erikson, the son of Erik the Red (a famous Viking outlaw and explorer in his own right), was born in either 970 or 980, depending on which historian you believe. His own family, though, did not raise Leif, which was a Viking tradition. Instead, one of Erik's prisoners taught Leif reading and writing, languages, sailing, and weaponry. At age 12, Leif was considered a man and returned to his family. He killed a man during a dispute shortly after his return, and the council banished the Erikson clan to Greenland.

In 999, Leif left Greenland and traveled to Norway, where he would serve as a guard to King Olaf Tryggvason. It was there that he became a convert to Christianity. Leif later tried to return home with the intention of taking supplies and spreading Christianity to Greenland, but his ship was blown off course and he arrived in a strange new land: present-day Newfoundland, Canada.

When he finally returned to his adopted homeland of Greenland, Leif consulted with a merchant who had also seen the shores of this previously unknown land. The son of the legendary Viking explorer then gathered a crew of 35 men and set sail. Leif became the first European to set foot in the New World as he explored present-day Baffin Island and Labrador, Canada. His crew called the land Vinland since it was plentiful with grapes.

During their time in present-day Newfoundland, Leif's expedition made contact with the natives, whom they referred to as Skraelings (which translates to "wretched ones" in Norse). There are several secondhand accounts of their meetings. Some contemporaries described trade between the peoples. Other accounts describe clashes where the Skraelings defeated the Viking explorers with long spears, while still others claim the Vikings dominated the natives. Regardless of the circumstances, it seems that the Vikings made contact of some kind. This happened around 1000, nearly 500 years before Columbus famously sailed the ocean blue.

Eventually, in 1003, Leif set sail for home and arrived at Greenland with a ship full of timber.

In 1020, 17 years later, the legendary Viking died. Many believe that Leif Erikson should receive more credit for his contributions in exploring the New World.

1. Which of the following best describes how the author generally presents the information?
    a. Chronological order
    b. Comparison-contrast
    c. Cause-effect
    d. Conclusion-premises

2. Which of the following is an opinion, rather than a historical fact, expressed by the author?
   a. Leif Erikson was definitely the son of Erik the Red; however, historians debate the year of his birth.
   b. Leif Erikson's crew called the land Vinland since it was plentiful with grapes.
   c. Leif Erikson deserves more credit for his contributions in exploring the New World.
   d. Leif Erikson explored the Americas nearly 500 years before Christopher Columbus.

3. Which of the following most accurately describes the author's main conclusion?
   a. Leif Erikson is a legendary Viking explorer.
   b. Leif Erikson deserves more credit for exploring America hundreds of years before Columbus.
   c. Spreading Christianity motivated Leif Erikson's expeditions more than any other factor.
   d. Leif Erikson contacted the natives nearly five hundred years before Columbus.

4. Which of the following best describes the author's intent in the passage?
   a. To entertain
   b. To inform
   c. To alert
   d. To suggest

5. Which of the following can be logically inferred from the passage?
   a. The Vikings disliked exploring the New World.
   b. Leif Erikson's banishment from Iceland led to his exploration of present-day Canada.
   c. Leif Erikson never shared his stories of exploration with the King of Norway.
   d. Historians have difficulty definitively pinpointing events in the Vikings' history.

See answers on the next page.

Answer Explanations

1. D: The passage does not proceed in chronological order since it begins by pointing out Christopher Columbus's explorations in America, so Choice *A* does not work. Although the author compares and contrasts Erikson with Columbus, this is not the main way the information is presented; therefore, Choice *B* does not work. Choice *C* is also incorrect because there is no mention of or reference to cause and effect in the passage. However, the passage does offer a conclusion (Leif Erikson deserves more credit) and premises (first European to set foot in the New World and first to contact the natives) to substantiate Erikson's historical importance. Thus, Choice *D* is correct.

2. C: Choice *A* is wrong because it describes facts: Leif Erikson was the son of Erik the Red and historians debate Leif's date of birth. These are not opinions. Choice *B* is wrong; Erikson calling the land Vinland is a verifiable fact, as is Choice *D*, because he did contact the natives almost 500 years before Columbus. Choice *C* is the correct answer because it is the author's opinion that Erikson deserves more credit. Another person could argue that Columbus or another explorer deserves more credit, which makes it an opinion rather than a historical fact.

3. B: Choice *A* is wrong because the author aims to go beyond describing Erikson as merely a legendary Viking. Choice *C* is wrong because the author does not focus on Erikson's motivations, let alone name the spreading of Christianity as his primary objective. Although it's true that Erikson contacted the natives 500 years before Columbus, Choice *D* is wrong because it isn't the author's main conclusion, it is simply a fact used to support the main conclusion. Choice *B* is correct because it accurately identifies the author's statement that Erikson deserves more credit than he has received for being the first European to explore the New World.

4. B: Choice *B* is correct because the author wants the reader to be informed about Leif Erikson's contribution to exploring the new world. While several other answers are possible options, Choice *B* is the strongest. Choice *A* is incorrect because the author is not in any way trying to entertain the reader. Choice *C* is incorrect because the nature of the writing does not indicate the author would be satisfied with the reader merely being alerted to Erikson's exploration; instead, the author is making an argument about the credit he should receive. Choice *D* is incorrect because the author goes beyond merely a suggestion; suggest is too vague.

5. D: Choice *A* is wrong because the author never addresses the Vikings' state of mind or emotions. Choice *B* is wrong because the author does not elaborate on Erikson's exile and whether he would have become an explorer if not for his banishment. Choice *C* is wrong because there is not enough information to support this premise. It is unclear whether Erikson informed the King of Norway of his findings. Although it is true that the king did not send a follow-up expedition, he could have simply chosen not to expend the resources after receiving Erikson's news. It is not possible to logically infer whether Erikson told him. Choice *D* is correct because the uncertainty about Leif Erikson's birth year is an example of how historians have trouble pinning down important details in Viking history.

Writing

Expression of Ideas

The writing portion of the test is about *how* the information is communicated rather than the subject matter itself. The good news is there isn't any writing! Instead, it's like being an editor helping the writer find the best ways to express their ideas. Things to consider include: how well a topic is developed, how accurately facts are presented, whether the writing flows logically and cohesively, and how effectively the writer uses language. This can seem like a lot to remember, but these concepts are the same ones taught way back in elementary school.

One last thing to remember while going through this guide is not to be intimidated by the terminology. Phrases like "pronoun-antecedent agreement" and "possessive determiners" can sound confusing and complicated, but the ideas are often quite simple and easy to understand. Though proper terminology is used to explain the rules and guidelines, the writing portion of the Kaplan Admissions Test is not a technical grammar test.

Organization

Good writing is not merely a random collection of sentences. No matter how well written, sentences must relate and coordinate appropriately to one another. If not, the writing seems random, haphazard, and disorganized. Therefore, good writing must be *organized* (where each sentence fits a larger context and relates to the sentences around it).

Organizational Structure

Depending on the purpose of one's writing and the assignment given, the writer will need to select the most appropriate organizational structure for their work.

The following organizational structures are most common:

- **Problem/solution**—organized by an analysis/overview of a problem, followed by potential solution(s)
- **Cause/effect**—organized by the effects resulting from a cause or the cause(s) of a particular effect
- **Spatial order**—organized by points that suggest location or direction—e.g., top to bottom, right to left, outside to inside
- **Chronological/sequence order**—organized by points presented to indicate a passage of time or through purposeful steps/stages
- **Comparison/contrast**—organized by points that indicate similarities and/or differences between two things or concepts
- **Order of importance**—organized by priority of points, often most significant to least significant or vice versa

Transition Words

The writer should act as a guide, showing the reader how all the sentences fit together. Consider this example:

> Seat belts save more lives than any other automobile safety feature. Many studies show that airbags save lives as well. Not all cars have airbags. Many older cars don't. Air bags aren't entirely reliable. Studies show that in 15% of accidents, airbags don't deploy as designed. Seat belt malfunctions are extremely rare.

There's nothing wrong with any of these sentences individually, but together they're disjointed and difficult to follow. The best way for the writer to communicate information is through the use of **transition words**. Here are examples of transition words and phrases that tie sentences together, enabling a more natural flow:

- To show causality: *as a result, therefore,* and *consequently*
- To compare and contrast: *however, but*, and *on the other hand*
- To introduce examples: *for instance, namely*, and *including*
- To show order of importance: *foremost, primarily, secondly*, and *lastly*

The above is not a complete list of transitions. There are many more that can be used; however, most fit into these or similar categories. The important point is that the words should clearly show the relationship between sentences, supporting information, and the main idea.

Here is an update to the previous example using transition words. These changes make it easier to read and bring clarity to the writer's points:

> Seat belts save more lives than any other automobile safety feature. Many studies show that airbags save lives as well. However, not all cars have airbags. For instance, some older cars don't. Furthermore, air bags aren't entirely reliable. For example, studies show that in 15% of accidents, airbags don't deploy as designed. But, on the other hand, seat belt malfunctions are extremely rare.

Also be prepared to analyze whether the writer is using the best transition word or phrase for the situation. Take this sentence for example: "As a result, seat belt malfunctions are extremely rare." This sentence doesn't make sense in the context above because the writer is trying to show the *contrast* between seat belts and airbags, not the causality.

Logical Sequence

Even if the writer includes plenty of information to support their point, the writing is only effective when the information is in a logical order. **Logical sequencing** is really just common sense, but it's also an important writing technique. First, the writer should introduce the main idea, whether for a paragraph, a section, or the entire piece. Then they should present evidence to support the main idea by using transitional language. This shows the reader how the information relates to the main idea and to the sentences around it. The writer should then take time to interpret the information, making sure necessary connections are obvious to the reader. Finally, the writer can summarize the information in a closing section.

Although most writing follows this pattern, it isn't a set rule. Sometimes writers change the order for effect. For example, the writer can begin with a surprising piece of supporting information to grab the reader's attention, and then transition to the main idea. Thus, if a passage doesn't follow the logical order, don't immediately assume it's wrong. However, most writing usually settles into a logical sequence after a nontraditional beginning.

Focus

Good writing stays focused and on topic. During the test, determine the main idea for each passage and then look for times when the writer strays from the point they're trying to make. Let's go back to the seat belt example. If the writer suddenly begins talking about how well airbags, crumple zones, or other safety features work to save lives, they might be losing focus from the topic of "safety belts."

Focus can also refer to individual sentences. Sometimes the writer does address the main topic, but in a confusing way. For example:

> Thanks to seat belt usage, survival in serious car accidents has shown a consistently steady increase since the development of the retractable seat belt in the 1950s.

This statement is definitely on topic, but it's not easy to follow. A simpler, more focused version of this sentence might look like this:

> Seat belts have consistently prevented car fatalities since the 1950s.

Providing adequate information is another aspect of focused writing. Statements like "seat belts are important" and "many people drive cars" are true, but they're so general that they don't contribute much to the writer's case. When reading a passage, watch for these kinds of unfocused statements.

Introductions and Conclusions

Examining the writer's strategies for introductions and conclusions puts the reader in the right mindset to interpret the rest of the passage. Look for methods the writer might use for **introductions** such as:

- Stating the main point immediately, followed by outlining how the rest of the piece supports this claim.
- Establishing important, smaller pieces of the main idea first, and then grouping these points into a case for the main idea.
- Opening with a quotation, anecdote, question, seeming paradox, or other piece of interesting information, and then using it to lead to the main point.

Whatever method the writer chooses, the introduction should make their intention clear, establish their voice as a credible one, and encourage a person to continue reading.

Conclusions tend to follow a similar pattern. In them, the writer restates their main idea a final time, often after summarizing the smaller pieces of that idea. If the introduction uses a quote or anecdote to grab the reader's attention, the conclusion often makes reference to it again. Whatever way the writer chooses to arrange the conclusion, the final restatement of the main idea should be clear and simple for the reader to interpret.

Finally, conclusions shouldn't introduce any new information.

Precision

People often think of **precision** in terms of math, but precise word choice is another key to successful writing. Since language itself is imprecise, it's important for the writer to find the exact word or words to convey the full, intended meaning of a given situation. For example:

> The number of deaths has gone down since seat belt laws started.

There are several problems with this sentence. First, the word *deaths* is too general. From the context, it's assumed that the writer is referring only to *deaths* caused by car accidents. However, without clarification, the sentence lacks impact and is probably untrue. The phrase "gone down" might be accurate, but a more precise word could provide more information and greater accuracy. Did the numbers show a slow and steady decrease of highway fatalities or a sudden drop? If the latter is true, the writer is missing a chance to make their point more dramatically. Instead of "gone down" they could substitute *plummeted, fallen drastically*, or *rapidly diminished* to bring the information to life. Also, the phrase "seat belt laws" is unclear. Does it refer to laws requiring cars to include seat belts or to laws requiring drivers and passengers to use them? Finally, *started* is not a strong verb. Words like *enacted* or *adopted* are more direct and make the content more real. When put together, these changes create a far more powerful sentence:

> The number of highway fatalities has plummeted since laws requiring seat belt usage were enacted.

However, it's important to note that precise word choice can sometimes be taken too far. If the writer of the sentence above takes precision to an extreme, it might result in the following:

> The incidence of high-speed, automobile accident related fatalities has decreased 75% and continued to remain at historical lows since the initial set of federal legislations requiring seat belt use were enacted in 1992.

This sentence is extremely precise, but it takes so long to achieve that precision that it suffers from a lack of clarity. Precise writing is about finding the right balance between information and flow. This is also an issue of conciseness (discussed in the next section).

The last thing to consider with precision is a word choice that's not only unclear or uninteresting, but also confusing or misleading. For example:

> The number of highway fatalities has become hugely lower since laws requiring seat belt use were enacted.

In this case, the reader might be confused by the word *hugely*. Huge means large, but here the writer uses *hugely* to describe something small. Though most readers can decipher this, doing so disconnects them from the flow of the writing and makes the writer's point less effective.

Conciseness

"Less is more" is a good rule to follow when writing a sentence. Unfortunately, writers often include extra words and phrases that seem necessary at the time, but add nothing to the main idea. This confuses the reader and creates unnecessary repetition. Writing that lacks **conciseness** is usually guilty of excessive wordiness and redundant phrases. Here's an example containing both of these issues:

> When legislators decided to begin creating legislation making it mandatory for automobile drivers and passengers to make use of seat belts while in cars, a large number of them made those laws for reasons that were political reasons.

There are several empty or "fluff" words here that take up too much space. These can be eliminated while still maintaining the writer's meaning. For example:

- "decided to begin" could be shortened to "began"
- "making it mandatory for" could be shortened to "requiring"
- "make use of" could be shortened to "use"
- "a large number" could be shortened to "many"

In addition, there are several examples of redundancy that can be eliminated:

- "legislators decided to begin creating legislation" and "made those laws"
- "automobile drivers and passengers" and "while in cars"
- "reasons that were political reasons"

These changes are incorporated as follows:

> When legislators began requiring drivers and passengers to use seat belts, many of them did so for political reasons.

There are many examples of redundant phrases, such as "complete and total," "time schedule," and "transportation vehicle." If asked to identify a redundant phrase on the test, look for words that are close together with the same (or similar) meanings.

Proposition

The **proposition** (also called the **claim** since it can be true or false) is a clear statement of the point or idea the writer is trying to make. The length or format of a proposition can vary, but it often takes the form of a **topic sentence**. A good topic sentence is:

- Clear: does not weave a complicated web of words for the reader to decode or unwrap
- Concise: presents only the information needed to make the claim and doesn't clutter up the statement with unnecessary details
- Precise: clarifies the exact point the writer wants to make and doesn't use broad, overreaching statements

Look at the following example:

> The civil rights movement, from its genesis in the Emancipation Proclamation to its current struggles with de facto discrimination, has changed the face of the United States more than any other factor in its history.

Is the statement clear? Yes, the statement is fairly clear, although other words can be substituted for "genesis" and "de facto" to make it easier to understand.

Is the statement concise? No, the statement is not concise. Details about the Emancipation Proclamation and the current state of the movement are unnecessary for a topic sentence. Those details should be saved for the body of the text.

Is the statement precise? No, the statement is not precise. What exactly does the writer mean by "changed the face of the United States"? The writer should be more specific about the effects of the movement. Also, suggesting that something has a greater impact than anything else in U.S. history is far too ambitious a statement to make.

A better version might look like this:

> The civil rights movement has greatly increased the career opportunities available for Black Americans.

The unnecessary language and details are removed, and the claim can now be measured and supported.

Support

Once the main idea or proposition is stated, the writer attempts to prove or support the claim with text evidence and supporting details.

Take for example the sentence, "Seat belts save lives." Though most people can't argue with this statement, its impact on the reader is much greater when supported by additional content. The writer can support this idea by:

- Providing statistics on the rate of highway fatalities alongside statistics for estimated seat belt usage.
- Explaining the science behind a car accident and what happens to a passenger who doesn't use a seat belt.
- Offering anecdotal evidence or true stories from reliable sources on how seat belts prevent fatal injuries in car crashes.

However, using only one form of supporting evidence is not nearly as effective as using a variety to support a claim. Presenting only a list of statistics can be boring to the reader, but providing a true story that's both interesting and humanizing helps. In addition, one example isn't always enough to prove the writer's larger point, so combining it with other examples is extremely effective for the writing. Thus, when reading a passage, don't just look for a single form of supporting evidence.

Another key aspect of supporting evidence is a **reliable source**. Does the writer include the source of the information? If so, is the source well known and trustworthy? Is there a potential for bias? For example, a seat belt study done by a seat belt manufacturer may have its own agenda to promote.

Effective Language Use

Language can be analyzed in a variety of ways. But one of the primary ways is its effectiveness in communicating and especially convincing others.

Rhetoric is a literary technique used to make the writing (or speaking) more effective or persuasive. Rhetoric makes use of other effective language devices such as irony, metaphors, allusion, and repetition. An example of the rhetorical use of repetition would be: "Let go, I say, let go!!!".

Figures of Speech

A **figure of speech** (sometimes called an **idiom**) is a rhetorical device. It's a phrase that's not intended to be taken literally.

When the writer uses a figure of speech, their intention must be clear if it's to be used effectively. Some phrases can be interpreted in a number of ways, causing confusion for the reader. In the writing section, questions may ask for an alternative to a problematic word or phrase. Look for clues to the writer's true intention to determine the best replacement. Likewise, some figures of speech may seem out of place in a more formal piece of writing. To show this, here is the previous seat belt example but with one slight change:

> Seat belts save more lives than any other automobile safety feature. Many studies show that airbags save lives as well. However, not all cars have airbags. For instance, some older cars don't. In addition, air bags aren't entirely reliable. For example, studies show that in 15% of accidents, airbags don't deploy as designed. But, on the other hand, seat belt malfunctions happen once in a blue moon.

Most people know that "once in a blue moon" refers to something that rarely happens. However, because the rest of the paragraph is straightforward and direct, using this figurative phrase distracts the reader. In this example, the earlier version is much more effective.

Rhetorical Fallacies

A **rhetorical fallacy** is an argument that doesn't make sense. It usually involves distracting the reader from the issue at hand in some way. There are many kinds of rhetorical fallacies. Here are just a few, along with examples of each:

- **Ad Hominem**: Makes an irrelevant attack against the person making the claim, rather than addressing the claim itself.

  > Senator Wilson opposed the new seat belt legislation, but should we really listen to someone who's been divorced four times?

- **Exaggeration**: Represents an idea or person in an obviously excessive manner.

  > Senator Wilson opposed the new seat belt legislation. Maybe she thinks if more people die in car accidents, it will help with overpopulation.

- **Stereotyping (or Categorical Claim)**: Claims that all people of a certain group are the same in some way.

  > Senator Wilson still opposes the new seat belt legislation. You know women can never admit when they're wrong.

When examining a possible rhetorical fallacy, carefully consider the point the writer is trying to make and if the argument directly relates to that point. If something feels wrong, there's a good chance that a fallacy is at play. The writing portion of the test doesn't expect the fallacy to be named using specific terms like those above. However, questions can include identifying why something is a fallacy or suggesting a sounder argument.

Style, Tone, and Mood

Style, tone, and mood are often thought to be the same thing. Though they're closely related, there are important differences to keep in mind. The easiest way to do this is to remember that style "creates and affects" tone and mood. More specifically, style is *how the writer uses words* to create the desired tone and mood for their writing.

Style

Style can include any number of technical writing choices, and some may have to be analyzed on the test. A few examples of style choices include:

- Sentence Construction: When presenting facts, does the writer use shorter sentences to create a quicker sense of the supporting evidence, or do they use longer sentences to elaborate and explain the information?
- Technical Language: Does the writer use jargon to demonstrate their expertise in the subject, or do they use ordinary language to help the reader understand things in simple terms?
- Formal Language: Does the writer refrain from using contractions such as *won't* or *can't* to create a more formal tone, or do they use a colloquial, conversational style to connect to the reader?
- Formatting: Does the writer use a series of shorter paragraphs to help the reader follow a line of argument, or do they use longer paragraphs to examine an issue in great detail and demonstrate their knowledge of the topic?

On the test, examine the writer's style and how their writing choices affect the way the passage comes across.

Tone

As previously mentioned, **tone** refers to the writer's attitude toward the subject matter. When analyzing tone, consider what the writer is trying to achieve in the passage, and how they *create* the tone using style.

Mood

Mood refers to the feelings and atmosphere that the writer's words create for the reader. Like tone, many nonfiction pieces can have a neutral mood. To return to the previous example, if the writer would choose to include information about a person they know being killed in a car accident, the passage would suddenly carry an emotional component that is absent in the previous examples. Depending on how they present the information, the writer can create a sad, angry, or even hopeful mood. When analyzing the mood, consider what the writer wants to accomplish and whether the best choice was made to achieve that end.

Consistency

Whatever style, tone, and mood the writer uses, good writing should remain **consistent** throughout. If the writer chooses to include the tragic, personal experience above, it would affect the style, tone, and mood of the entire piece. It would seem out of place for such an example to be used in the middle of a neutral, measured, and analytical piece. To adjust the rest of the piece, the writer needs to make additional choices to remain consistent. For example, the writer might decide to use the word *tragedy* in place of the more neutral *fatality*, or they could describe a series of car-related deaths as an *epidemic*. Adverbs and adjectives such as *devastating* or *horribly* could be included to maintain this consistent attitude toward the content. When analyzing writing, look for sudden shifts in style, tone, and mood, and consider whether the writer would be wiser to maintain the prevailing strategy.

Syntax

Syntax is the order of words in a sentence. While most of the writing on the test has proper syntax, there may be questions on ways to vary the syntax for effectiveness. One of the easiest writing mistakes to spot is repetitive sentence structure. For example:

> Seat belts are important. They save lives. People don't like to use them. We have to pass seat belt laws. Then more people will wear seat belts. More lives will be saved.

What's the first thing that comes to mind when reading this example? The short, choppy, and repetitive sentences! In fact, most people notice this syntax issue more than the content itself. By combining some sentences and changing the syntax of others, the writer can create a more effective writing passage:

> Seat belts are important because they save lives. Since people don't like to use seat belts, though, more laws requiring their usage need to be passed. Only then will more people wear them and only then will more lives be saved.

Many rhetorical devices can be used to vary syntax (more than can possibly be named here). These often have intimidating names like *anadiplosis*, *metastasis*, and *paremptosis*. The test questions don't ask for definitions of these tricky techniques, but they can ask how the writer plays with the words and what effect that has on the writing. For example, *anadiplosis* is when the last word (or phrase) from a sentence is used to begin the next sentence:

> Cars are driven by people. People cause accidents. Accidents cost taxpayers money.

The test doesn't ask for this technique by name, but be prepared to recognize what the writer is doing and why they're using the technique in this situation. In this example, the writer is probably using *anadiplosis* to demonstrate causation.

Logical Comparison

Writers often make comparisons in their writing. However, it's easy to make mistakes in sentences that involve comparisons, and those mistakes are difficult to spot. Try to find the error in the following sentence:

> Senator Wilson's proposed seat belt legislation was similar to Senator Abernathy.

Can't find it? First, ask what two things are actually being compared. It seems like the writer *wants* to compare two different types of legislation, but the sentence actually compares legislation ("Senator Wilson's proposed seat belt legislation") to a person ("Senator Abernathy"). This is a strange and illogical comparison to make.

So how can the writer correct this mistake? The answer is to make sure that the second half of the sentence logically refers back to the first half. The most obvious way to do this is to repeat words:

> Senator Wilson's proposed seat belt legislation was similar to Senator Abernathy's seat belt legislation.

Now the sentence is logically correct, but it's a little wordy and awkward. A better solution is to eliminate the word-for-word repetition by using suitable replacement words:

> Senator Wilson's proposed seat belt legislation was similar to that of Senator Abernathy.

> Senator Wilson's proposed seat belt legislation was similar to the bill offered by Senator Abernathy.

Here's another similar example:

> More lives in the U.S. are saved by seat belts than Japan.

The writer probably means to compare lives saved by seat belts in the U.S. to lives saved by seat belts in Japan. Unfortunately, the sentence's meaning is garbled by an illogical comparison, and instead refers to U.S. lives saved *by Japan* rather than *in Japan.* To resolve this issue, first repeat the words and phrases needed to make an identical comparison:

> More lives in the U.S. are saved by seat belts than lives in Japan are saved by seat belts.

Then, use a replacement word to clean up the repetitive text:

> More lives in the U.S. are saved by seat belts than in Japan.

Parts of Speech

Nouns

A **common noun** is a word that identifies any of a class of people, places, or things. Examples include numbers, objects, animals, feelings, concepts, qualities, and actions. *A, an,* or *the* usually precedes the common noun. These parts of speech are called **articles**. Here are some examples of sentences using nouns preceded by articles.

> *A* building is under construction.

> *The* girl would like to move to *the* city.

An **abstract noun** is an idea, state, or quality. It is something that can't be touched, such as happiness, courage, evil, or humor.

A **proper noun** (also called a **proper name**) is used for the specific name of an individual person, place, or organization. The first letter in a proper noun is capitalized. "My name is *Mary*." "I work for *Walmart*."

Nouns sometimes serve as adjectives (which themselves describe nouns), such as "hockey player" and "state government."

Pronouns

A word used in place of a noun is known as a **pronoun**. Pronouns are words like *I, mine, hers,* and *us*.

Pronouns can be split into different classifications (as shown below) which make them easier to learn; however, it's not important to memorize the classifications.

- **Personal pronouns**: refer to people
- **First person pronouns**: *we, I, our, mine*
- **Second person pronouns:** *you, yours*
- **Third person pronouns:** *he, she, they, them, it*
- **Possessive pronouns**: demonstrate ownership (*mine, his, hers, its, ours, theirs, yours)*
- **Interrogative pronouns**: ask questions (*what, which, who, whom, whose*)
- **Relative pronouns**: include the five interrogative pronouns and others that are relative (*whoever, whomever, that, when, where*)
- **Demonstrative pronouns**: replace something specific (*this, that, those, these*)
- **Reciprocal pronouns**: indicate something was done or given in return (*each other, one another*)
- **Indefinite pronouns**: have a nonspecific status (*anybody, whoever, someone, everybody, somebody*)

Indefinite pronouns such as *anybody, whoever, someone, everybody*, and *somebody* command a singular verb form, but others such as *all, none,* and *some* could require a singular or plural verb form.

Antecedents

An **antecedent** is the noun to which a pronoun refers; it needs to be written or spoken before the pronoun is used. For many pronouns, antecedents are imperative for clarity. In particular, a lot of the personal, possessive, and demonstrative pronouns need antecedents. Otherwise, it would be unclear who or what someone is referring to when they use a pronoun like *he* or *this*.

Pronoun reference means that the pronoun should refer clearly to one, clear, unmistakable noun (the antecedent).

Pronoun-antecedent agreement refers to the need for the antecedent and the corresponding pronoun to agree in gender, person, and number. Here are some examples:

> The *kidneys* (plural antecedent) are part of the urinary system. *They* (plural pronoun) serve several roles.

> The kidneys are part of the *urinary system* (singular antecedent). *It* (singular pronoun) is also known as the renal system.

Pronoun Cases

The **subjective pronouns** —*I, you, he/she/it, we, they,* and *who*—are the subjects of the sentence.

Example: *They* have a new house.

The **objective pronouns**—*me, you* (*singular*), *him/her, us, them,* and *whom*—are used when something is being done for or given to someone; they are objects of the action.

Example: The teacher has an apple for *us*.

The **possessive pronouns**—*mine, my, your, yours, his, hers, its, their, theirs, our,* and *ours*—are used to denote that something (or someone) belongs to someone (or something).

Example: It's *their* chocolate cake.

Even Better Example: It's *my* chocolate cake!

One of the greatest challenges and worst abuses of pronouns concerns *who* and *whom*. Just knowing the following rule can eliminate confusion. *Who* is a subjective-case pronoun used only as a subject or subject complement. *Whom* is only objective-case and, therefore, the object of the verb or preposition.

Who is going to the concert?

You are going to the concert with *whom*?

Hint: When using *who* or *whom*, think of whether someone would say *he* or *him*. If the answer is *he*, use *who*. If the answer is *him*, use *whom*. This trick is easy to remember because *he* and *who* both end in vowels, and *him* and *whom* both end in the letter *M*.

Many possessive pronouns sound like contractions. For example, many people get *it's* and *its* confused. The word *it's* is the contraction for *it is*. The word *its* without an apostrophe is the possessive form of *it*.

I love that wooden desk. It's beautiful. (contraction)

I love that wooden desk. Its glossy finish is beautiful. (possessive)

If you are not sure which version to use, replace *it's/its* with *it is* and see if that sounds correct. If so, use the contraction (*it's*). That trick also works for *who's/whose, you're/your*, and *they're/their*.

Adjectives

"The *extraordinary* brain is the *main* organ of the central nervous system." The adjective *extraordinary* describes the brain in a way that causes one to realize it is more exceptional than some of the other organs while the adjective *main* defines the brain's importance in its system.

An **adjective** is a word or phrase that names an attribute that describes or clarifies a noun or pronoun. This helps the reader visualize and understand the characteristics—size, shape, age, color, origin, etc.—of a person, place, or thing that otherwise might not be known. Adjectives breathe life, color, and depth into the subjects they define. Life would be *drab* and *colorless* without adjectives!

Adjectives often precede the nouns they describe.

> *She drove her* new *car.*

However, adjectives can also come later in the sentence.

> *Her car is* new*.*

Adjectives using the prefix *a*– can only be used after a verb.

> Correct: The dog was alive until the car ran up on the curb and hit him.

> Incorrect: The alive dog was hit by a car that ran up on the curb.

Other examples of this rule include *awake, ablaze, ajar, alike,* and *asleep*.

Other adjectives used after verbs concern states of health.

> The girl was finally *well* after a long bout of pneumonia.

> The boy was *fine* after the accident.

An adjective phrase is not a bunch of adjectives strung together, but a group of words that describes a noun or pronoun and, thus, functions as an adjective. *Very happy* is an adjective phrase; so are *way too hungry* and *passionate about traveling.*

Possessives

In grammar, **possessive nouns** and **possessive pronouns** show ownership.

Singular nouns are generally made possessive with an apostrophe and an *s* (*'s*).

> My *uncle's* new car is silver.

> The *dog's* bowl is empty.

> *James's* ties are becoming outdated.

Plural nouns ending in *s* are generally made possessive by just adding an apostrophe (*'*):

> The pistachio nuts' saltiness is added during roasting. (The saltiness of pistachio nuts is added during roasting.)

> The students' achievement tests are difficult. (The achievement tests of the students are difficult.)

If the plural noun does not end in an *s* such as *women,* then it is made possessive by adding an *apostrophe s* (*'s*)—*women's.*

Possessive pronouns can be first person (*mine*), second person (*yours*), or third person (*theirs*).

Indefinite possessive pronouns such as *nobody* or *someone* become possessive by adding an *apostrophe s— nobody's* or *someone's.*

Verbs

A verb is the part of speech that describes an action, state of being, or occurrence.

A verb forms the main part of a predicate of a sentence. This means that the verb explains what the noun (which will be discussed shortly) is doing. A simple example is *time flies*. The verb *flies* explains what the action of the noun, *time*, is doing. This example is a **main verb**.

Helping (auxiliary) verbs are words like *have, do, be, can, may, should, must,* and *will.* "I *should* go to the store." Helping verbs assist main verbs in expressing tense, ability, possibility, permission, or obligation.

Particles are minor function words like *not, in, out, up,* or *down* that become part of the verb itself. "I might *not*."

Participles are words formed from verbs that are often used to modify a noun, noun phrase, verb, or verb phrase.

> The *running* teenager collided with the cyclist.

Participles can also create compound verb forms.

> He *is speaking*.

Participial phrases are made up of the participle and modifiers, complements, or objects.

> *Crying for most of an hour*, the baby didn't seem to want to nap.
>
> *Having already taken this course*, the student was bored during class.

Verbs have five basic forms: the **base** form, the **-*s*** form, the ***-ing*** form, the **past** form, and the **past participle** form.

The past forms are either **regular** (*love/loved; hate/hated*) or **irregular** because they don't end by adding the common past tense suffix "-ed" (*go/went; fall/fell; set/set*).

Adverbs

Adverbs have more functions than adjectives because they modify or qualify verbs, adjectives, or other adverbs as well as word groups that express a relation of place, time, circumstance, or cause. Therefore, adverbs answer any of the following questions: *How, when, where, why, in what way, how often, how much, in what condition,* and/or *to what degree. How good looking is he? He is very handsome.*

Here are some examples of adverbs for different situations:

- how: quickly
- when: daily
- where: there
- in what way: easily
- how often: often
- how much: much
- in what condition: badly
- what degree: hardly

As one can see, for some reason, many adverbs end in *-ly.*

Adverbs do things like emphasize (*really, simply,* and *so*), amplify (*heartily, completely,* and *positively*), and tone down (*almost, somewhat,* and *mildly*).

Adverbs also come in phrases.

> The dog ran as <u>though his life depended on it.</u>

Prepositions

Prepositions are connecting words and, while there are only about 150 of them, they are used more often than any other individual groups of words. They describe relationships between other words. They are placed before a noun or pronoun, forming a phrase that modifies another word in the sentence. **Prepositional phrases** begin with a preposition and end with a noun or pronoun, the **object of the preposition**. *A pristine lake is <u>near the store</u> and <u>behind the bank</u>.*

Some commonly used prepositions are *about, after, anti, around, as, at, behind, beside, by, for, from, in, into, of, off, on, to,* and *with.*

Complex prepositions, which also come before a noun or pronoun, consist of two or three words such as *according to, in regards to,* and *because of.*

Interjections

Interjections are words used to express emotion. Examples include *wow*, *ouch*, and *hooray*. Interjections are often separate from sentences; in those cases, the interjection is directly followed by an exclamation point. In other cases, the interjection is included in a sentence and followed by a comma. The punctuation plays a big role in the intensity of the emotion that the interjection is expressing. Using a comma or semicolon indicates less excitement than using an exclamation mark.

Conjunctions

Conjunctions are vital words that connect words, phrases, thoughts, and ideas. Conjunctions show relationships between components. There are two types:

Coordinating conjunctions are the primary class of conjunctions placed between words, phrases, clauses, and sentences that are of equal grammatical rank; the coordinating conjunctions are *for, and, nor, but, or, yet,* and *so*. A useful memorization trick is to remember that all the first letters of these conjunctions collectively spell the word fanboys.

> I need to go shopping, *but* I must be careful to leave enough money in the bank.

> She wore a black, red, *and* white shirt.

Subordinating conjunctions are the secondary class of conjunctions. They connect two unequal parts, one **main** (or **independent**) and the other **subordinate** (or **dependent**). I must go to the store *even though* I do not have enough money in the bank.

> *Because* I read the review, I do not want to go to the movie.

Notice that the presence of subordinating conjunctions makes clauses dependent. *I read the review* is an independent clause, but *because* makes the clause dependent. Thus, it needs an independent clause to complete the sentence.

Sentences

First, let's review the basic elements of sentences.

A **sentence** is a set of words that make up a grammatical unit. The words must have certain elements and be spoken or written in a specific order to constitute a complete sentence that makes sense.

1. A sentence must have a **subject** (a noun or noun phrase). The subject tells whom or what the sentence is addressing (i.e., what it is about).

2. A sentence must have an **action** or **state of being** (a verb). To reiterate: A verb forms the main part of the predicate of a sentence. This means that it explains what the noun is doing.

3. A sentence must convey a complete thought.

When examining writing, be mindful of grammar, structure, spelling, and patterns. Sentences can come in varying sizes and shapes; so, the point of grammatical correctness is not to stamp out creativity or diversity in writing. Rather, grammatical correctness ensures that writing will be enjoyable and clear. One of the most common methods for catching errors is to mouth the words as you read them. Many typos are fixed automatically by our brain, but mouthing the words often circumvents this instinct and helps one read what's actually on the page. Often, grammar errors are caught not by memorization of grammar rules but by the training of one's mind to know whether something *sounds* right or not.

Types of Sentences

There isn't an overabundance of absolutes in grammar, but here is one: every sentence in the English language falls into one of four categories.

- Declarative: a simple statement that ends with a period

  The price of milk per gallon is the same as the price of gasoline.

- Imperative: a command, instruction, or request that ends with a period

  Buy milk when you stop to fill up your car with gas.

- Interrogative: a question that ends with a question mark

  Will you buy the milk?

- Exclamatory: a statement or command that expresses emotions like anger, urgency, or surprise and ends with an exclamation mark

  Buy the milk now!

Declarative sentences are the most common type, probably because they are comprised of the most general content, without any of the bells and whistles that the other three types contain. They are, simply, declarations or statements of any degree of seriousness, importance, or information.

Imperative sentences often seem to be missing a subject. The subject is there, though; it is just not visible or audible because it is *implied*. Look at the imperative example sentence.

Buy the milk when you fill up your car with gas.

You is the implied subject, the one to whom the command is issued. This is sometimes called *the understood you* because it is understood that *you* is the subject of the sentence.

Interrogative sentences—those that ask questions—are defined as such from the idea of the word *interrogation*, the action of questions being asked of suspects by investigators. Although that is serious business, interrogative sentences apply to all kinds of questions.

To exclaim is at the root of **exclamatory sentences**. These are made with strong emotions behind them. The only technical difference between a declarative or imperative sentence and an exclamatory one is the exclamation mark at the end. The example declarative and imperative sentences can both become an exclamatory one simply by putting an exclamation mark at the end of the sentences.

The price of milk per gallon is the same as the price of gasoline!

Buy milk when you stop to fill up your car with gas!

After all, someone might be really excited by the price of gas or milk, or they could be mad at the person that will be buying the milk! However, as stated before, exclamation marks in abundance defeat their own purpose! After a while, they begin to cause fatigue! When used only for their intended purpose, they can have their expected and desired effect.

Independent and Dependent Clauses

Independent and dependent clauses are strings of words that contain both a subject and a verb. An **independent clause** can stand alone as complete thought, but a **dependent clause** cannot. A dependent clause relies on other words to be a complete sentence.

Independent clause: The keys are on the counter.

Dependent clause: If the keys are on the counter

Notice that both clauses have a subject (*keys*) and a verb (*are*). The independent clause expresses a complete thought, but the word *if* at the beginning of the dependent clause makes it *dependent* on other words to be a complete thought.

Independent clause: If the keys are on the counter, please give them to me.

This example constitutes a complete sentence since it includes at least one verb and one subject and is a complete thought. In this case, the independent clause has two subjects (*keys* & an implied *you*) and two verbs (*are* & *give*).

Independent clause: I went to the store.

Dependent clause: Because we are out of milk,

Complete Sentence: Because we are out of milk, I went to the store.

Complete Sentence: I went to the store because we are out of milk.

Sentence Structures

A **simple sentence** has one independent clause.

I am going to win.

A **compound sentence** has two independent clauses. A conjunction—*for, and, nor, but, or, yet, so*—links them together. Note that each of the independent clauses has a subject and a verb.

I am going to win, but the odds are against me.

A **complex sentence** has one independent clause and one or more dependent clauses.

I am going to win, even though I don't deserve it.

Even though I don't deserve it is a dependent clause. It does not stand on its own. Some conjunctions that link an independent and a dependent clause are *although*, *because*, *before*, *after*, *that*, *when*, *which*, and *while*.

A **compound-complex sentence** has at least three clauses, two of which are independent and at least one that is a dependent clause.

While trying to dance, I tripped over my partner's feet, but I regained my balance quickly.

The dependent clause is *While trying to dance*.

Run-Ons and Fragments

Run-Ons

A common mistake in writing is the run-on sentence. A **run-on** is created when two or more independent clauses are joined without the use of a conjunction, a semicolon, a colon, or a dash. We don't want to use commas where periods belong. Here is an example of a run-on sentence:

Making wedding cakes can take many hours I am very impatient, I want to see them completed right away.

There are a variety of ways to correct a run-on sentence. The method you choose will depend on the context of the sentence and how it fits with neighboring sentences:

Making wedding cakes can take many hours. I am very impatient. I want to see them completed right away. (Use periods to create more than one sentence.)

Making wedding cakes can take many hours; I am very impatient—I want to see them completed right away. (Correct the sentence using a semicolon, colon, or dash.)

Making wedding cakes can take many hours, and I am very impatient and want to see them completed right away. (Correct the sentence using coordinating conjunctions.)

I am very impatient because I would rather see completed wedding cakes right away than wait for it to take many hours. (Correct the sentence by revising.)

Fragments

Remember that a complete sentence must have both a subject and a verb. Complete sentences consist of at least one independent clause. Incomplete sentences are called **sentence fragments**. A sentence fragment is a common error in writing. Sentence fragments can be independent clauses that start with subordinating words, such as *but, as, so that,* or *because,* or they could simply be missing a subject or verb.

A fragment error can be corrected by adding the fragment to a nearby sentence or by adding or removing words to make it an independent clause. For example:

Dogs are my favorite animals. Because cats are too lazy. (Incorrect; the word *because* creates a sentence fragment)

Dogs are my favorite animals because cats are too lazy. (Correct; this is a dependent clause.)

Dogs are my favorite animals. Cats are too lazy. (Correct; this is a simple sentence.)

Subject and Predicate

Every complete sentence can be divided into two parts: the subject and the predicate.

Subjects: Subjects are needed in sentences to tell the reader who or what the sentence describes. Subjects can be simple or complete, and they can be direct or indirect. There can also be compound subjects.

Simple subjects are the noun or pronouns the sentence describes, without modifiers. The simple subject can come before or after the verb in the sentence:

The big brown <u>dog</u> is the calmest one.

Complete subjects are the subject together with all of its describing words or modifiers.

The <u>big brown dog</u> is the calmest one. (The complete subject is big brown dog.)

Direct subjects are subjects that appear in the text of the sentence, as in the example above. **Indirect subjects** are implied. The subject is "you," but the word *you* does not appear.

Indirect subjects are usually in imperative sentences that issue a command or order:

Feed the short skinny dog first. (The understood *you* is the subject.)

Watch out—he's really hungry! (The sentence warns *you* to watch out.)

Compound subjects occur when two or more nouns join together to form a plural subject.

<u>Carson</u> and <u>Emily</u> make a great couple.

Predicates: Once we have identified the subject of the sentence, the rest of the sentence becomes the predicate. Predicates are formed by the verb, the direct object, and all words related to it.

We went to see the Cirque du' Soleil performance.

The gigantic green character was funnier than all the rest.

A **predicate nominative** renames the subject:

John is a carpenter.

A **predicate adjective** describes the subject:

Margaret is beautiful.

Direct objects are the nouns in the sentence that are receiving the action. Sentences don't necessarily need objects. Sentences only need a subject and a verb.

The clown brought the acrobat the hula-hoop. (What is being brought? the hula-hoop)

Then he gave the trick pony a soapy bath. (What is being given? a soapy bath)

Indirect objects are words that tell us to or for whom or what the action is being done. For there to be an indirect object, there first must always be a direct object.

The clown brought the acrobat the hula-hoop. (Who is getting the direct object? the acrobat)
Then he gave the trick pony a soapy bath. (What is getting the bath? the trick pony)

Phrases

A **phrase** is a group of words that do not make a complete thought or a clause. They are parts of sentences or clauses. Phrases can be used as nouns, adjectives, or adverbs. A phrase does not contain both a subject and a verb.

Prepositional Phrases

A **prepositional phrase** shows the relationship between a word in the sentence and the object of the preposition. The object of the preposition is a noun that follows the preposition.

The orange pillows are on the couch.

On is the preposition, and *couch* is the object of the preposition.

She brought her friend with the nice car.

With is the preposition, and *car* is the object of the preposition. Here are some common prepositions:

about	as	at	after
by	for	from	in
of	on	to	with

Verbals and Verbal Phrases

Verbals are forms of verbs that act as other parts of speech. They can be used as nouns, adjectives, or adverbs. Though they are verb forms, they are not to be used as the verb in the sentence. A word group that is based on a verbal is considered a **verbal phrase**. There are three major types of verbals: participles, gerunds, and infinitives.

Participles are verbals that act as adjectives. The present participle ends in *–ing*, and the past participle ends in *–d*, *-ed*, *-n*, or *-t*.

Verb	Present Participle	Past Participle
walk	walking	walked
share	sharing	shared

Participial phrases are made up of the participle and modifiers, complements, or objects.

> Crying for most of an hour, the baby didn't seem to want to nap.
>
> Having already taken this course, the student was bored during class.
>
> *Crying for most of an hour* and *Having already taken this course* are the participial phrases.

Gerunds are verbals that are used as nouns and end in *–ing*. A gerund can be the subject or object of the sentence like a noun. Note that a present participle can also end in *–ing*, so it is important to distinguish between the two. The gerund is used as a noun, while the participle is used as an adjective.

> Swimming is my favorite sport.
>
> I wish I were sleeping.

A **gerund phrase** includes the gerund and any modifiers or complements, direct objects, indirect objects, or pronouns.

> Cleaning the house is my least favorite weekend activity.

Cleaning the house is the gerund phrase acting as the subject of the sentence.

> The most important goal this year is raising money for charity.

Raising money for charity is the gerund phrase acting as the direct object.

> The police accused the woman of stealing the car.

The gerund phrase *stealing the car* is the object of the preposition in this sentence.

An **infinitive** is a verbal made up of the word *to* and a verb. Infinitives can be used as nouns, adjectives, or adverbs.

> Examples: *To eat, to jump, to swim, to lie, to call, to work*

An **infinitive phrase** is made up of the infinitive plus any complements or modifiers. The infinitive phrase *to wait* is used as the subject in this sentence:

To wait was not what I had in mind.

The infinitive phrase *to sing* is used as the subject complement in this sentence:

Her dream is to sing.

The infinitive phrase *to grow* is used as an adverb in this sentence:

Children must eat to grow.

Appositive Phrases

An **appositive** is a noun or noun phrase that renames a noun that comes immediately before it in the sentence. An appositive can be a single word or several words. These phrases can be essential or nonessential. An **essential appositive phrase** is necessary to the meaning of the sentence and a **nonessential appositive phrase** is not. It is important to be able to distinguish these for purposes of comma use.

Essential: My sister Christina works at a school.

Naming which sister is essential to the meaning of the sentence, so no commas are needed.

Nonessential: My sister, who is a teacher, is coming over for dinner tonight.

Who is a teacher is not essential to the meaning of the sentence, so commas are required.

Absolute Phrases

An **absolute phrase** modifies a noun without using a conjunction. It is not the subject of the sentence and is not a complete thought on its own. Absolute phrases are set off from the independent clause with a comma.

Arms outstretched, she yelled at the sky.

All things considered, this has been a great day.

Subject-Verb Agreement

The subject of a sentence and its verb must agree. The cornerstone rule of **subject-verb agreement** is that subject and verb must agree in number. Whether the subject is singular or plural, the verb must follow suit.

Incorrect: The houses is new.

Correct: The houses are new.

Also Correct: The house is new.

In other words, a singular subject requires a singular verb; a plural subject requires a plural verb.

The words or phrases that come between the subject and verb do not alter this rule.

Incorrect: The houses built of brick is new.

Correct: The houses built of brick are new.

Incorrect: The houses with the sturdy porches is new.

Correct: The houses with the sturdy porches are new.

The subject will always follow the verb when a sentence begins with *here* or *there.* Identify these with care.

Incorrect: Here *is* the *houses* with sturdy porches.

Correct: Here *are* the *houses* with sturdy porches.

The subject in the sentences above is not *here*, it is *houses*. Remember, *here* and *there* are never subjects. Be careful that contractions such as *here's* or *there're* do not cause confusion!

Two subjects joined by *and* require a plural verb form, except when the two combine to make one thing:

Incorrect: Garrett and Jonathan is over there.

Correct: Garrett and Jonathan are over there.

Incorrect: Spaghetti and meatballs are a delicious meal!

Correct: Spaghetti and meatballs is a delicious meal!

In the example above, *spaghetti and meatballs* is a compound noun. However, *Garrett and Jonathan* is not a compound noun.

Two singular subjects joined by *or, either/or,* or *neither/nor* call for a singular verb form.

Incorrect: Butter or syrup are acceptable.

Correct: Butter or syrup is acceptable.

Plural subjects joined by *or*, *either/or*, or *neither/nor* are, indeed, plural.

The chairs or the boxes are being moved next.

If one subject is singular and the other is plural, the verb should agree with the closest noun.

Correct: The chair or the boxes are being moved next.

Correct: The chairs or the box is being moved next.

Some plurals of money, distance, and time call for a singular verb.

Incorrect: Three dollars *are* enough to buy that.

Correct: Three dollars *is* enough to buy that.

For words declaring degrees of quantity such as *many of, some of,* or *most of,* let the noun that follows *of* be the guide:

Incorrect: Many of the books is in the shelf.

Correct: Many of the books are in the shelf.

Incorrect: Most of the pie *are* on the table.

Correct: Most of the pie *is* on the table.

For indefinite pronouns like *anybody* or *everybody*, use singular verbs.

Everybody *is* going to the store.

However, the pronouns *few, many, several, all, some,* and *both* have their own rules and use plural forms.

Some *are* ready.

Some nouns like *crowd* and *congress* are called **collective nouns** and they require a singular verb form.

Congress *is* in session.

The news *is* over.

Books and movie titles, though, including plural nouns such as *Great Expectations*, also require a singular verb. Remember that only the subject affects the verb. While writing tricky subject-verb arrangements, say them aloud. Listen to them. Once the rules have been learned, one's ear will become sensitive to them, making it easier to pick out what's right and what's wrong.

Dangling and Misplaced Modifiers

A **modifier** is a word or phrase meant to describe or clarify another word in the sentence. When a sentence has a modifier but is missing the word it describes or clarifies, it's an error called a **dangling modifier**. We can fix the sentence by revising to include the word that is being modified. Consider the following examples with the modifier underlined:

Incorrect: Having walked five miles, this bench will be the place to rest. (This implies that the bench walked the miles, not the person.)

Correct: Having walked five miles, Matt will rest on this bench. (*Having walked five miles* correctly modifies *Matt*, who did the walking.)

Incorrect: Since midnight, my dreams have been pleasant and comforting. (The adverb clause *since midnight* cannot modify the noun *dreams*.)

Correct: Since midnight, I have had pleasant and comforting dreams. (*Since midnight* modifies the verb have had, telling us when the dreams occurred.)

Sometimes the modifier is not located close enough to the word it modifies for the sentence to be clearly understood. In this case, we call the error a **misplaced modifier**. Here is an example with the modifier underlined.

> Incorrect: We gave the hot cocoa to the children that was filled with marshmallows. (This sentence implies that the children are what are filled with marshmallows.)
>
> Correct: We gave the hot cocoa that was filled with marshmallows to the children. (The cocoa is filled with marshmallows. The modifier is near the word it modifies.)

Split Infinitives

An **infinitive** is made up of the word *to* and a verb, such as: **to run, to jump, to ask**. A **split infinitive** is created when a word comes between *to* and the verb.

> Split infinitive: To quickly run
>
> Correction: To run quickly
>
> Split infinitive: To quietly ask
>
> Correction: To ask quietly

Double Negatives

A **double negative** is a negative statement that includes two negative elements. This is incorrect in Standard English.

> Incorrect: She hasn't never come to my house to visit.
>
> Correct: She has never come to my house to visit.

The intended meaning is that she has never come to the house, so the double negative is incorrect. However, it is possible to use two negatives to create a positive statement.

> Correct: She was not unhappy with her performance on the quiz.

In this case, the double negative*, was not unhappy*, is intended to show a positive, so it is correct. This means that she was somewhat happy with her performance.

Parallel Structure in a Sentence

Parallel structure, also known as **parallelism**, refers to using the same grammatical form within a sentence. This is important in lists and for other components of sentences.

> Incorrect: At the recital, the boys and girls were dancing, singing, and played musical instruments.
>
> Correct: At the recital, the boys and girls were dancing, singing, and playing musical instruments.

Notice that in the second example, *played* is not in the same verb tense as the other verbs, nor is it compatible with the helping verb *were*. To test for parallel structure in lists, try reading each item as if it were the only item in the list.

> The boys and girls were dancing.
>
> The boys and girls were singing.
>
> The boys and girls were played musical instruments.

Suddenly, the error in the sentence becomes very clear. Here's another example:

> Incorrect: After the accident, I informed the police *that Mrs. Holmes backed* into my car, *that Mrs. Holmes got out* of her car to look at the damage, and *she was driving* off without leaving a note.
>
> Correct: After the accident, I informed the police *that Mrs. Holmes backed* into my car, *that Mrs. Holmes got out* of her car to look at the damage, and *that Mrs. Holmes drove off* without leaving a note.
>
> Correct: After the accident, I informed the police that Mrs. Holmes *backed* into my car, *got out* of her car to look at the damage, and *drove off* without leaving a note.

Note that there are two ways to fix the nonparallel structure of the first sentence. The key to parallelism is consistent structure.

Punctuation

Commas

A **comma** (,) is the punctuation mark that signifies a pause—breath—between parts of a sentence. It denotes a break of flow. As with so many aspects of writing structure, authors will benefit by memorizing all of the different ways in which commas can be used so as not to abuse them.

In a complex sentence—one that contains a subordinate (dependent) clause or clauses—the use of a comma is dictated by where the subordinate clause is located. If the subordinate clause is located before the main clause, a comma is needed between the two clauses.

> I will not pay for the steak, *because I don't have that much money*.

Generally, if the subordinate clause is placed after the main clause, no punctuation is needed.

> I did well on my exam because I studied two hours the night before.

Notice how the last clause is dependent because it earlier independent clauses to make sense.

Use a comma on both sides of an interrupting phrase.

> I will pay for the ice cream, *chocolate and vanilla*, and then will eat it all myself.

The words forming the phrase in italics are nonessential (extra) information. To determine if a phrase is nonessential, try reading the sentence without the phrase and see if it's still coherent.

A comma is not necessary in this next sentence because no interruption—nonessential or extra information—has occurred. Read sentences aloud when uncertain.

> I will pay for his chocolate and vanilla ice cream and then will eat it all myself.

If the nonessential phrase comes at the beginning of a sentence, a comma should only go at the end of the phrase. If the phrase comes at the end of a sentence, a comma should only go at the beginning of the phrase.

Other types of interruptions include the following:

- Interjections: Oh no, I am not going.
- Abbreviations: Barry Potter, M.D., specializes in heart disorders.
- Direct addresses: Yes, Claudia, I am tired and going to bed.
- Parenthetical phrases: His wife, lovely as she was, was not helpful.
- Transitional phrases: Also, it is not possible.

The second comma in the following sentence is called an **Oxford comma**.

> I will pay for ice cream, syrup, and pop.

It is a comma used after the second-to-last item in a series of three or more items. It comes before the word *or* or *and*. Not everyone uses the Oxford comma; it is optional, but many believe it is needed. The comma functions as a tool to reduce confusion in writing. So, if omitting the Oxford comma would cause confusion, then it's best to include it.

Commas are used in math to mark the place of thousands in numerals, breaking them up so they are easier to read. Other uses for commas are in dates (*March 19, 2016*), letter greetings (*Dear Sally,*), and in between cities and states (*Louisville, KY*).

Apostrophes

This punctuation mark, the **apostrophe** ('), is a versatile little mark. It has a few different functions:

- Quotes: Apostrophes are used when a second quote is needed within a quote.

    > In my letter to my friend, I wrote, "The girl had to get a new purse, and guess what Mary did? She said, 'I'd like to go with you to the store.' I knew Mary would buy it for her."

- Contractions: Another use for an apostrophe in the quote above is a contraction. *I'd* is used for *I would.*

    The basic rule for making contractions is one area of spelling that is pretty straightforward: combine the two words by inserting an apostrophe (') in the space where a letter is omitted. For example, to combine *you* and *are*, drop the *a* and put the apostrophe in its place: *you're*.

    > he + is = he's
    >
    > you + all = y'all (informal but often misspelled)

- Possession: An apostrophe followed by the letter *s* shows possession (*Mary's* purse). If the possessive word is plural, the apostrophe generally just follows the word.

- The trees' leaves are all over the ground.

Ellipses

An ellipsis (...) is used to show that there is more to the quoted text than is necessary for the current discussion. Writers use them in place of words, lines, phrases, list content, or paragraphs that might just as easily have been omitted from a passage of writing. This can be done to save space or to focus only on the specifically relevant material.

> Exercise is good for some unexpected reasons. Watkins writes, "Exercise has many benefits such as...reducing cancer risk."

In the example above, the ellipsis takes the place of the other benefits of exercise that are more expected.

The ellipsis may also be used to show a pause in sentence flow.

> "I'm wondering...how this could happen," Dylan said in a soft voice.

Semicolons

The **semicolon** (;) might be described as a heavy-handed comma. Take a look at these two examples:

> I will pay for the ice cream, but I will not pay for the steak.
>
> I will pay for the ice cream; I will not pay for the steak.

What's the difference? The first example has a comma and a conjunction separating the two independent clauses. The second example does not have a conjunction, but there are two independent clauses in the sentence, so something more than a comma is required. In this case, a semicolon is used.

Two independent clauses can only be joined in a sentence by either a comma and conjunction or a semicolon. If one of those tools is not used, the sentence will be a run-on. Remember that while the clauses are independent, they need to be closely related in order to be contained in one sentence.

Another use for the semicolon is to separate items in a list when the items themselves require commas.

> The family lived in Phoenix, Arizona; Oklahoma City, Oklahoma; and Raleigh, North Carolina.

Colons

Colons (:) have many miscellaneous functions. Colons can be used to precede further information or a list. In these cases, a colon should only follow an independent clause. Here are some examples:

> Humans take in sensory information through five basic senses: sight, hearing, smell, touch, and taste.
>
> The meal includes the following components:
>
> - Caesar salad
> - spaghetti

- garlic bread
- cake

Colons can also be used to introduce an appositive.

> The family got what they needed: a reliable vehicle.

While a comma is more common, a colon can also precede a formal quotation.

> He said to the crowd: "Let's begin!"

The colon is used after the greeting in a formal letter.

> Dear Sir:

> To Whom It May Concern:

In the writing of time, the colon separates the minutes from the hour (*4:45 p.m.*). The colon can also be used to indicate a ratio between two numbers (*50:1*).

Hyphens

The **hyphen** (-) is a small dash mark that can be used to join words to show that they are linked.

Hyphens can connect two words that work together as a single adjective (a compound adjective).

> honey-covered biscuits

Some words always require hyphens even if not serving as an adjective.

> merry-go-round

Hyphens always go after certain prefixes like *anti-* & *all-*.

Hyphens should also be used when the absence of the hyphen would cause a strange vowel combination (*semi-engineer*) or confusion. For example, *re-collect* should be used to describe something being gathered twice rather than being written as *recollect*, which means to remember.

Parentheses and Dashes

Parentheses are half-round brackets that look like this: *( )*. They set off a word, phrase, or sentence that is an afterthought, explanation, or side note relevant to the surrounding text but not essential. A pair of commas is often used to set off this sort of information, but parentheses are generally used for information that would not fit well within a sentence or that the writer deems not important enough to be structurally part of the sentence.

> The picture of the heart (see above) shows the major parts you should memorize.

> Mount Everest is one of three mountains in the world that are over 28,000 feet high (K2 and Kanchenjunga are the other two).

See how the sentences above are complete without the parenthetical statements? In the first example, *see above* would not have fit well within the flow of the sentence. The second parenthetical statement could have been a separate sentence, but the writer deemed the information not pertinent to the topic.

The **em-dash** (—) is a mark longer than a hyphen used as a punctuation mark in sentences and to set apart a relevant thought. Even after plucking out the line separated by the dash marks, the sentence will be intact and make sense.

> Looking out the airplane window at the landmarks—Lake Clarke, Thompson Community College, and the bridge—she couldn't help but feel excited to be home.

The dashes use is similar to that of parentheses or a pair of commas. So, what's the difference? Many believe that using dashes makes the clause within them stand out while using parentheses is subtler. It's advised to not use dashes when commas could be used instead.

Quotation Marks

Quotation marks ("") are used in a number of ways. Here are some instances where quotation marks should be used:

- To indicate a quote that was taken from somewhere else, either from a verbal or written source
- Dialogue for characters in narratives. When characters speak, the first word should always be capitalized, and the punctuation goes inside the quotes. For example:

  > Janie said, "The tree fell on my car during the hurricane."

- Around titles of songs, short stories, essays, and chapters in books
- To emphasize a certain word
- To refer to a word as the word itself

Capitalization

Here's a non-exhaustive list of things that should be capitalized:

- The first word of every sentence
- The first letter of proper nouns (World War II)
- Holidays (Valentine's Day)
- The days of the week and months of the year (Tuesday, March)
- The first word, last word, and all major words in the titles of books, movies, songs, and other creative works (In the novel, *To Kill a Mockingbird*, note that *a* is lowercase since it's not a major word, but *to* is capitalized since it's the first word of the title.)
- Titles when preceding a proper noun (President Roberto Gonzales, Aunt Judy)

When simply using a word such as president or secretary, though, the word is not capitalized.

> Officers of the new business must include a *president* and *treasurer*.

Seasons—*spring, fall*, etc.—are not capitalized.

North, *south*, *east*, and *west* are capitalized when referring to regions but are not when being used for directions. In general, if it's preceded by *the* it should be capitalized.

> I'm from the South.
> I drove south.

Various Homonyms

That/Which

The pronouns that and which are both used to refer to nouns—but they are not interchangeable. The rule is to use the word *that* in essential clauses and phrases that help convey the meaning of the sentence. Use the word *which* in nonessential (less important) clauses. Typically, *which* clauses are enclosed in commas.

> The morning that I fell asleep in class caused me a lot of trouble.

> This morning's coffee, which had too much creamer, woke me up.

Who/Whom

We use the pronouns *who* and *whom* to refer to people. We always use *who* when it is the subject of the sentence or clause. *Whom* is always the object of a verb or preposition.

> Who hit the baseball for the home run? (subject)

> The baseball fell into the glove of whom? (object of the preposition of)

> The umpire called whom "out"? (object of the verb called)

To/Too/Two

to: a preposition or infinitive (*to walk, to run, walk to the store, run to the tree*)
too: means also, as well, or very (*She likes cookies, too.*; *I ate too much.*)
two: a number (*I have two cookies. She walked to the store two times.*)

There/Their/They're

there: an adjective, adverb, or pronoun used to start a sentence or indicate place (*There are four vintage cars over there.*)
their: a possessive pronoun used to indicate belonging (*Their car is the blue and white one.*)
they're: a contraction of the words "they are" (*They're going to enter the vintage car show.*)

Your/You're

your: a possessive pronoun (*Your artwork is terrific.*)
you're: a contraction of the words "you are" (*You're a terrific artist.*)

Its/It's

its: a possessive pronoun (*The elephant had its trunk in the water.*)
it's: a contraction of the words "it is" (*It's an impressive animal.*)

Affect/Effect

affect: as a verb means "to influence" (*How will the earthquake affect your home?*); as a noun means "emotion or mood" (*Her affect was somber.*)
effect: as a verb means "to bring about" (*She will effect a change through philanthropy.*); as a noun means "a result of" (*The effect of the earthquake was devastating.*)

Other mix-ups: Other pairs of words cause mix-ups but are not necessarily homonyms. Here are a few of those:

Bring/Take

bring: when the action is coming toward (*Bring me the money.*)
take: when the action is going away from (*Take her the money.*)

Can/May

can: means "able to" (*The child can ride a bike.*)
may: asks permission (*The child asked if he may ride his bike.*)

Than/Then

than: a conjunction used for comparison (*I like tacos better than pizza.*)
then: an adverb telling when something happened (*I ate and then slept.*)

Disinterested/Uninterested

disinterested: used to mean "neutral" (*The jury remains disinterested during the trial.*)
uninterested: used to mean "bored" (*I was uninterested during the lecture.*)

Percent/Percentage

percent: used when there is a number involved (*Five percent of us like tacos.*)
percentage: used when there is no number (*That is a low percentage.*)

Fewer/Less

fewer: used for things you can count (*He has fewer playing cards.*)
less: used for things you cannot count, as well as time (*He has less talent. You have less than a minute.*)

Farther/Further

farther: used when discussing distance (*His paper airplane flew farther than mine.*)
further: used to mean "more" (*He needed further information.*)

Lend/Loan

lend: a verb used for borrowing (*Lend me your lawn mower. He will lend it to me.*)
loan: a noun used for something borrowed (*She applied for a student loan.*)

Note

Some people have problems with these:

- regardless/irregardless
- a lot/alot

Irregardless and *alot* are always incorrect. Don't use them.

Please keep in mind that grammar questions on the actual exam may be hospital related.

Final Tips

Usage Conventions

On the test, don't overlook simple, obvious writing errors such as these:

- Is the first word in a sentence capitalized?
- Are countries, geographical features, and proper nouns capitalized?
- Conversely, are words capitalized that should *not* be?
- Do sentences end with proper punctuation marks?
- Are commas and quotation marks used appropriately?
- Do contractions include apostrophes?
- Are apostrophes used for plurals? (Almost never!)

Look for Context

Keep in mind that the test may give several choices to replace a writing selection, and all of them may be grammatically correct. In such cases, choose the answer that makes the most sense in the context of the piece. What's the writer trying to say? What's their main idea? Look for the answer that best supports this theme.

Use Your Instincts

With the few notable exceptions above, instinct is often the best guide to spotting writing problems. If something sounds wrong, then it may very well be wrong. The good thing about a test like this is that the problem doesn't have to be labeled as an example of "faulty parallelism" or "improper noun-pronoun agreement." It's enough just to recognize that a problem exists and choose the best solution.

Take a Break

After reading and thinking about all of these aspects of grammar so intensely, the brain may start shutting down. If the words aren't making sense, or reading the same sentence several times still has no meaning, it's time to stop. Take a thirty-second vacation. Forget about grammar, syntax, and writing for half a minute to clear the mind. Take a few deep breaths and think about something to do after the test is over. It's surprising how quickly the brain refreshes itself!

Practice Quiz

The next five questions are based on the following passage:

> [1]Since the first discovery of dinosaur bones, scientists has made strides in technological development and methodologies used to investigate these extinct animals. [2]We know more about dinosaurs than ever before and are still learning, fascinating new things about how they looked and lived. [3]However, one has to ask, how if earlier perceptions of dinosaurs continue to influence people's understanding of these creatures? [4] Can these perceptions inhibit our progress towards further understanding dinosaurs?
>
> [5]The biggest problem with studying dinosaurs is simply that there are no living dinosaurs to observe. [6]All discoveries associated with these animals are based on physical remains. [7]To gauge behavioral characteristics, scientists cross-examine these finds with living animals to explore potential similarities. [8]While this method is effective, these are still deductions. [9] For example, a Spinosaurus has a large sail, or a finlike structure, that grows from its back. [10]Paleontologists know this sail exists and have ideas for its function however, they are uncertain of which idea is the true function. [11]Some scientists believe the sail serves to regulate the Spinosaurus' body temperature and yet others believe its used to attract mates. [12]Still other scientists think the sail was used to intimidate other predatory dinosaurs for self-defense. [13]These are all viable explanations, but they are also influenced by what scientists know about modern animals. [14]Yet it's quite possible that the sail could hold a completely unique function.

1. Which sentence contains a subject-verb agreement error?
   a. Sentence 1
   b. Sentence 2
   c. Sentence 3
   d. Sentence 5

2. Where should the following sentence be inserted to make the most sense and aid the flow of the paragraph?
   Some ideas about dinosaurs can't be tested and confirmed simply because humans can't replicate a living dinosaur.

   a. Before Sentence 8
   b. Before Sentence 9
   c. Before Sentence 13
   d. Before Sentence 14

3. Which sentence contains an unnecessary or incorrect comma?
   a. Sentence 1
   b. Sentence 2
   c. Sentence 3
   d. Sentence 13

4. Which sentence is missing a semicolon?

a. Sentence 2
b. Sentence 3
c. Sentence 10
d. Sentence 13

5. Which sentence has made a mistake with a homophone?
a. Sentence 9
b. Sentence 10
c. Sentence 11
d. Sentence 14

See answers on the next page.

Answer Explanations

1. A: Sentence 1 contains a subject-verb agreement area because the singular has does not match the plural scientists. The sentence should read: Since the first discovery of dinosaur bones, scientists have made strides in technological development and methodologies used to investigate these extinct animals.

2. B: Of the choices given, this sentence would be best inserted before Sentence 9. As the paragraph stands now, there's a strange jump between Sentence 8 and 9 because Sentence 9 isn't giving an example of what is stated in Sentence 8, although it starts with "For example." The missing sentence (Some ideas about dinosaurs can't be tested and confirmed simply because humans can't replicate a living dinosaur) is what the example in Sentence 9 pertains to.

3. B: Sentence 2 has an unnecessary comma after learning: We know more about dinosaurs than ever before and are still learning, fascinating new things about how they looked and lived. The text after the comma is not a full dependent phrase or independent phrase with a conjunction. Therefore, it is inappropriately placed.

4. C: The sentence is a run-on as written. It needs a semicolon before however to correct this issue. Paleontologists know this sail exists and have ideas for is function; however, they are uncertain of which idea is the true function. This correction correctly applies a semicolon to introduce a new line of thought while remaining in a single sentence.

5. C: Sentence 11 has an issue with the homophone its/it's. As written, the sentence incorrectly uses its, which is possessive, when it needs it's, which is a contraction of it is. Some scientists believe the sail serves to regulate the Spinosaurus' body temperature and yet others believe it's (or it is) used to attract mates.

Mathematics

Numbers represent a quantity of objects. They function as placeholders for a value. Numbers can be better understood by their type and related characteristics.

Definitions

A few definitions:

Whole numbers: a set of numbers that does not contain any fractions or decimals. The set of whole numbers includes zero.

Example: 0, 1, 2, 3, 4, 189, 293 are all whole numbers.

Integers: whole numbers and their negative counterparts. (Zero does not have a negative counterpart here. Instead, zero is its own negative.)

Example: -1, -2, -3, -4, -5, 0, 1, 2, 3, 4, 5 are all integers.

-1, -2, -3, -4, -5 are considered negative integers, and 1, 2, 3, 4, 5 are considered positive integers.

Absolute value: describes the value of a number regardless of its sign. The symbol for absolute value is | |.

Example: The absolute value of 24 is 24 or |24| = 24.

The absolute value of -693 is 693 or |-693| = 693.

Even numbers: describes any number that can be divided by 2 evenly, meaning the answer has no decimal or remainder portion.

Example: 2, 4, 9,082, -2, -16, -504 are all considered even numbers, because they can be divided by 2, without leaving a remainder or forming a decimal. It does not matter whether the number is positive or negative.

Odd numbers: describes any number that does not divide evenly by 2.

Example: 1, 21, 541, 3,003, -9, -63, -1,257 are all considered odd numbers, because they cannot be divided by 2 without a remainder or a decimal.

Prime numbers: describes a number that is only evenly divisible, resulting in no remainder or decimal, by 1 and itself.

Example: 2, 3, 7, 13, 113 are all considered prime numbers because each can only be evenly divided by 1 and itself.

Composite numbers: describes a positive integer that is formed by multiplying two smaller integers together. Composite numbers can be divided evenly by numbers other than 1 or itself.

Example: 9, 24, 45, 66, 2,348, 10,002 are all considered composite numbers because they are the result of multiplying two smaller integers together.

Decimals: designated by a decimal point which indicates that what follows the point is a value that is less than 1 and is added to the integer number preceding the decimal point. The digit immediately following the decimal point is in the tenths place, the digit following the tenths place is in the hundredths place, and so on.

For example, the decimal number 1.735 has a value greater than 1 but less than 2. The 7 represents seven tenths of the unit 1 (0.7 or $\frac{7}{10}$); the 3 represents three hundredths of 1 (0.03 or $\frac{3}{100}$); and the 5 represents five thousandths of 1 (0.005 or $\frac{5}{1,000}$).

Real numbers: describes rational numbers and irrational numbers.

Rational numbers: describes any number that can be expressed as a fraction, with a non-zero denominator. Since any integer can be written with 1 in the denominator without changing its value, all integers are considered rational numbers. Every rational number has a decimal expression that terminates or repeats. That is, any rational number either will have a countable number of nonzero digits or will end with an ellipsis or a bar (3.6666... or $3.\bar{6}$) to depict repeating decimal digits. Some examples of rational numbers include 12, -3.54, $110.\overline{256}$, $\frac{-35}{10}$, and $4.\bar{7}$.

Irrational numbers: describes numbers that cannot be written as a finite or repeating decimal. Pi (π) is considered to be an irrational number because its decimal portion is unending or a non-repeating decimal. Pi (π) is the most common irrational number, but there are other well-known irrational numbers like e and $\sqrt{2}$.

Basic Operations with Whole Numbers

Addition

Addition is the combination of two numbers; their quantities are added together cumulatively. The sign for an addition operation is the + symbol. For example, $9 + 6 = 15$. The 9 and 6 combine to achieve a cumulative value, called a **sum**.

Addition follows the Commutative Property, which means that the order of the numbers in an addition equation can be switched without altering the result. The formula for the commutative property is $a + b = b + a$. Let's look at a few examples to see how the commutative property works:

$$7 = 3 + 4 = 4 + 3 = 7$$

$$20 = 12 + 8 = 8 + 12 = 20$$

Addition also follows the **Associative Property**, which means that the grouping of numbers doesn't matter in an addition problem. In other words, the presence or absence of parentheses is irrelevant. The formula for the associative property is $(a + b) + c = a + (b + c)$. Here are some examples of the associative property at work:

$$30 = (6 + 14) + 10 = 6 + (14 + 10) = 30$$

$$35 = 8 + (2 + 25) = (8 + 2) + 25 = 35$$

There are set columns for addition: ones, tens, hundreds, thousands, ten-thousands, hundred-thousands, millions, and so on. To add how many units there are total, each column needs to be combined, starting from the right, or the ones column.

THOUSANDS	HUNDREDS	TENS	ONES

Every 10 units in the ones column equals one in the tens column, and every 10 units in the tens column equals one in the hundreds column, and so on.

Example: The number 5,432 has 2 ones, 3 tens, 4 hundreds, and 5 thousands. The number 371 has 3 hundreds, 7 tens and 1 one. To combine, or add, these two numbers, simply add up how many units of each column exist. The best way to do this is by lining up the columns:

$$\begin{array}{r} 5\,4\,3\,2 \\ +\quad 3\,7\,1 \\ \hline \end{array}$$

The ones column adds $2 + 1$ for a total (sum) of 3.

The tens column adds $3 + 7$ for a total of 10; since 10 of that unit was collected, add 1 to the hundreds column to denote the total in the next column:

$$\begin{array}{r} 1 \\ 5\,4\,3\,2 \\ +\quad 3\,7\,1 \\ \hline 0\,3 \end{array}$$

When adding the hundreds column, this extra 1 needs to be combined, so it would be the sum of 4, 3, and 1.

$$4 + 3 + 1 = 8$$

The last, or thousands, column listed would be the sum of 5. Since there are no other numbers in this column, that is the final total.

The answer would look as follows:

$$\begin{array}{r} 5\,4\,3\,2 \\ +\quad 3\,7\,1 \\ \hline 5\,8\,0\,3 \end{array}$$

Example: Find the sum of 9,734 and 895.

Set up the problem:

$$\begin{array}{r} 9\,7\,3\,4 \\ +\quad 8\,9\,5 \\ \hline \end{array}$$

Total the columns:

$$\begin{array}{r} 9\,7\,3\,4 \\ +\quad 8\,9\,5 \\ \hline 1\,0\,6\,2\,9 \end{array}$$

In this example, another column (ten-thousands) is added to the left of the thousands column, to denote a carryover of 10 units in the thousands column. The final sum is 10,629.

When adding using all negative integers, the total is negative. The integers are simply added together and the negative symbol is tacked on.

$$(-12) + (-435) = -447$$

Subtraction

Subtraction is taking away one number from another, so their quantities are reduced. The sign designating a subtraction operation is the – symbol, and the result is called the **difference**. For example, $9 - 6 = 3$. The number *6* detracts from the number *9* to reach the difference *3*.

Unlike addition, subtraction follows neither the commutative nor associative properties. The order and grouping in subtraction impact the result.

$$15 = 22 - 7 \neq 7 - 22 = -15$$

$$3 = (10 - 5) - 2 \neq 10 - (5 - 2) = 7$$

When working through subtraction problems involving larger numbers, it's necessary to regroup the numbers. Let's work through a practice problem using regrouping:

$$\begin{array}{r} 3\,2\,5 \\ -\ \ 7\,7 \\ \hline \end{array}$$

Here, it is clear that the ones and tens columns for 77 are greater than the ones and tens columns for 325. To subtract this number, borrow from the tens and hundreds columns. When borrowing from a column, subtracting 1 from the lender column will add 10 to the borrower column:

$$\begin{array}{rrr} 3\text{-}1 & 10\text{+}2\text{-}1 & 10\text{+}5 \\ - & 7 & 7 \\ \hline \end{array} = \begin{array}{rrr} 2 & 11 & 15 \\ - & 7 & 7 \\ \hline 2 & 4 & 8 \end{array}$$

After ensuring that each digit in the top row is greater than the digit in the corresponding bottom row, subtraction can proceed as normal, and the answer is found to be 248.

Multiplication

Multiplication involves adding together multiple copies of a number. It is indicated by an $\times$ symbol or a number immediately outside of a parenthesis. For example:

$$5(8-2)$$

The two numbers being multiplied together are called **factors**, and their result is called a **product**. For example, $9 \times 6 = 54$. This can be shown alternatively by expansion of either the 9 or the 6:

$$9 \times 6 = 9 + 9 + 9 + 9 + 9 + 9 = 54$$

$$9 \times 6 = 6 + 6 + 6 + 6 + 6 + 6 + 6 + 6 + 6 = 54$$

Like addition, multiplication holds the commutative and associative properties:

$$115 = 23 \times 5 = 5 \times 23 = 115$$

$$84 = 3 \times (7 \times 4) = (3 \times 7) \times 4 = 84$$

Multiplication also follows the **distributive property**, which allows the multiplication to be distributed through parentheses. The formula for distribution is $a \times (b + c) = ab + ac$. This is clear after the examples:

$$45 = 5 \times 9 = 5(3 + 6) = (5 \times 3) + (5 \times 6) = 15 + 30 = 45$$

$$20 = 4 \times 5 = 4(10 - 5) = (4 \times 10) - (4 \times 5) = 40 - 20 = 20$$

If they have the same number of digits, select one for the top and one for the bottom. Line up the problem, and begin by multiplying the far-right column on the top and the far-right column on the bottom. If the answer to a column is more than 9, the ones place digit will be written below that column and the tens place digit will carry to the top of the next column to be added after those digits are multiplied. Write the answer below that column. Move to the next column to the left on the top, and multiply it by the same far right column on the bottom. Keep moving to the left one column at a time on the top number until the end.

Example:

Multiply 37×8

Line up the numbers, placing the one with the most digits on top.

$$\begin{array}{r} 3\ 7 \\ \times \quad 8 \\ \hline \end{array}$$

Multiply the far-right column on the top with the far-right column on the bottom (7×8). Write the answer, 56, as below: The ones value, 6, gets recorded, the tens value, 5, is carried.

$$\begin{array}{rrr} & {\scriptstyle +5} & \\ & 3 & 7 \\ \text{X} & & 8 \\ \hline & & 6 \end{array}$$

Move to the next column left on the top number and multiply with the far-right bottom (3×8). Remember to add any carry over after multiplying: $3 \times 8 = 24$, $24 + 5 = 29$. Since there are no more digits on top, write the entire number below.

$$\begin{array}{rrr} & {\scriptstyle +5} & \\ & 3 & 7 \\ \text{X} & & 8 \\ \hline 2 & 9 & 6 \end{array}$$

The solution is 296.

If there is more than one column to the bottom number, move to the row below the first strand of answers, mark a zero in the far-right column, and then begin the multiplication process again with the far-right column on top and the second column from the right on the bottom. For each digit in the bottom number, there will be a row of answers, each padded with the respective number of zeros on the right. Finally, add up all of the answer rows for one total number.

Example: Multiply 512×36.

Line up the numbers (the one with the most digits on top) to multiply.

Begin with the right column on top and the right column on bottom (2×6).

$$\begin{array}{rrrr} & 5 & 1 & 2 \\ \text{X} & & 3 & 6 \\ \hline \end{array}$$

Move one column left on top and multiply by the far-right column on the bottom (1×6). Add the carry over after multiplying: $1 \times 6 = 6$, $6 + 1 = 7$.

$$\begin{array}{rrrr} & & {\scriptstyle +1} & \\ & 5 & 1 & 2 \\ \text{x} & & 3 & 6 \\ \hline & & 7 & 2 \end{array}$$

Move one column left on top and multiply by the far-right column on the bottom (5×6). Since this is the last digit on top, write the whole answer below.

$$\begin{array}{r} 5\ 1\ 2 \\ \text{X}\quad 3\ 6 \\ \hline 3\ 0\ 7\ 2 \end{array}$$

Now move on to the second column on the bottom number. Starting on the far-right column on the top, repeat this pattern for the next number left on the bottom (2×3). Write the answers below the first line of answers; remember to begin with a zero placeholder on the far right.

$$\begin{array}{r} 5\ 1\ 2 \\ \text{X}\quad 3\ 6 \\ \hline 3\ 0\ 7\ 2 \\ 6\ 0 \end{array}$$

Continue the pattern (1×3).

$$\begin{array}{r} 5\ 1\ 2 \\ \text{X}\quad 3\ 6 \\ \hline 3\ 0\ 7\ 2 \\ 3\ 6\ 0 \end{array}$$

Since this is the last digit on top, write the whole answer below.

$$\begin{array}{r} 5\ 1\ 2 \\ \text{x}\quad 3\ 6 \\ \hline 3\ 0\ 7\ 2 \\ 1\ 5\ 3\ 6\ 0 \end{array}$$

Now add the answer rows together. Pay attention to ensure they are aligned correctly.

$$\begin{array}{r} 5\ 1\ 2 \\ \text{x}\quad 3\ 6 \\ \hline 3\ 0\ 7\ 2 \\ 1\ 5\ 3\ 6\ 0 \\ \hline 1\ 8\ 4\ 3\ 2 \end{array}$$

The solution is 18,432.

Division

Division and multiplication are inverses of each other in the same way that addition and subtraction are opposites. The signs designating a division operation are the $\div$ and / symbols. In division, the second number divides into the first.

The number before the division sign is called the **dividend** or, if expressed as a fraction, the numerator. For example, in $a \div b$, a is the dividend, while in $\frac{a}{b}$, a is the numerator.

The number after the division sign is called the **divisor** or, if expressed as a fraction, the denominator. For example, in $a \div b$, b is the divisor, while in $\frac{a}{b}$, b is the denominator.

Like subtraction, division doesn't follow the commutative property, as it matters which number comes before the division sign, and division doesn't follow the associative or distributive properties for the same reason. For example:

$$\frac{3}{2} = 9 \div 6 \neq 6 \div 9 = \frac{2}{3}$$

$$2 = 10 \div 5 = (30 \div 3) \div 5 \neq 30 \div (3 \div 5) = 30 \div \frac{3}{5} = 50$$

$$25 = 20 + 5 = (40 \div 2) + (40 \div 8) \neq 40 \div (2 + 8) = 40 \div 10 = 4$$

The answer to a division problem is called the **quotient**. If a divisor doesn't divide into a dividend evenly, whatever is left over is termed the **remainder**. The remainder can be further divided out into decimal form by using long division; however, this doesn't always give a quotient with a finite number of decimal places, so the remainder can also be expressed as a fraction over the original divisor.

Example:

Divide 1,050 by 42: $\frac{1{,}050}{42}$ or $1{,}050 \div 42$.

Set up the problem with the denominator being divided into the numerator.

$$42\overline{)\,1050}$$

Check for divisibility into the first unit of the numerator, 1.

42 cannot go into 1, so add on the next unit in the denominator, 0.

42 cannot go into 10, so add on the next unit in the denominator, 5.

42 can be divided into 105 two times. Write the 2 over the 5 in 105 and multiply 42×2. Write the 84 under 105 for subtraction and note the remainder, 21 is less than 42.

$$\begin{array}{r} 2 \\ 42\overline{)\,1050} \\ -84 \\ \hline 21 \end{array}$$

Drop the next digit in the numerator down to the remainder (making 21 into 210) to create a number 42 can divide into. 42 divides into 210 five times. Write the 5 over the 0 and multiply 42×5.

$$\begin{array}{r} 25 \\ 42\overline{)\,1050} \\ -84 \\ \hline 210 \end{array}$$

Write the 210 under 210 for subtraction. The remainder is 0.

$$\begin{array}{r} 25 \\ 42\overline{)1050} \\ -84 \\ \hline 210 \\ -210 \\ \hline 0 \end{array}$$

The solution is 25.

Example:

Divide 375 by 4: $\frac{375}{4}$ or $375 \div 4$.

Set up the problem.

$$4\overline{)375}$$

4 cannot divide into 3, so add the next unit from the numerator, 7. 4 divides into 37 nine times, so write the 9 above the 7. Multiply $4 \times 9 = 36$. Write the 36 under the 37 for subtraction. The remainder is 1 (1 is less than 4).

$$\begin{array}{r} 9 \\ 4\overline{)375} \\ -36 \\ \hline 1 \end{array}$$

Drop the next digit in the numerator, 5, making the remainder 15. 4 divides into 15, three times, so write the 3 above the 5. Multiply 4×3. Write the 12 under the 15 for subtraction, remainder is 3 (3 is less than 4).

$$\begin{array}{r} 93 \\ 4\overline{)375} \\ -36 \\ \hline 15 \\ -12 \\ \hline 3 \end{array}$$

The solution is 93 remainder 3 or 93 ¾ (the remainder can be written over the original denominator).

Positive and Negative Numbers

Signs

Aside from 0, numbers can be either positive or negative. The sign for a positive number is the plus sign or the + symbol, while the sign for a negative number is the minus sign or the – symbol. If a number has no designation, then it's assumed to be positive.

Absolute Values

Both positive and negative numbers are valued according to their distance from 0. Look at this number line for +3 and -3:

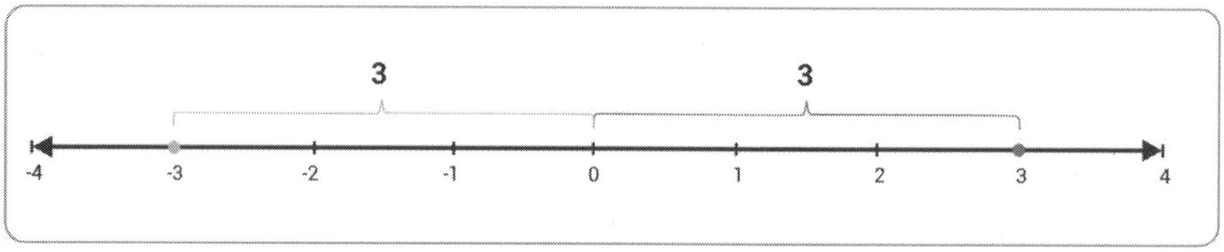

Both 3 and -3 are three spaces from 0. The distance from 0 is called its **absolute value**. Thus, both -3 and 3 have an absolute value of 3 since they're both three spaces away from 0.

An absolute number is written by placing | | around the number. So, $|3|$ and $|-3|$ both equal 3, as that's their common absolute value.

Implications for Addition and Subtraction

For addition, if all numbers are either positive or negative, simply add them together.

For example, $4 + 4 = 8$ and $-4 + -4 = -8$. However, things get tricky when some of the numbers are negative, and some are positive.

Take $6 + (-4)$ as an example. First, take the absolute values of the numbers, which are 6 and 4. Second, subtract the smaller value from the larger. The equation becomes $6 - 4 = 2$. Third, place the sign of the original larger number on the sum. Here, 6 is the larger number, and it's positive, so the sum is 2.

Here's an example where the negative number has a larger absolute value: $(-6) + 4$. The first two steps are the same as the example above. However, on the third step, the negative sign must be placed on the sum, as the absolute value of (-6) is greater than 4. Thus, $-6 + 4 = -2$.

The absolute value of numbers implies that subtraction can be thought of as flipping the sign of the number following the subtraction sign and simply adding the two numbers. This means that subtracting a negative number will in fact be adding the positive absolute value of the negative number. Here are some examples:

$$-6 - 4 = -6 + -4 = -10$$

$$3 - -6 = 3 + 6 = 9$$

$$-3 - 2 = -3 + -2 = -5$$

Implications for Multiplication and Division

For multiplication and division, if both numbers are positive, then the product or quotient is always positive. If both numbers are negative, then the product or quotient is also positive. However, if the numbers have opposite signs, the product or quotient is always negative.

Simply put, the product in multiplication and quotient in division is always positive, unless the numbers have opposing signs, in which case it's negative. Here are some examples:

$$(-6) \times (-5) = 30$$

$$(-50) \div 10 = -5$$

$$8 \times |-7| = 56$$

$$(-48) \div (-6) = 8$$

If there are more than two numbers in a multiplication problem, then whether the product is positive or negative depends on the number of negative numbers in the problem. If there is an odd number of negatives, then the product is negative. If there is an even number of negative numbers, then the result is positive.

Here are some examples:

$$(-6) \times 5 \times (-2) \times (-4) = -240$$

$$(-6) \times 5 \times 2 \times (-4) = 240$$

Decimals

Decimals mark the separation between the whole portion and the fractional (or decimal) portion of a number. For example, 3.15 has 3 in the whole portion and 15 in the fractional or decimal portion. A number such as 645 is all whole, but there is still a decimal place. The decimal place in 645 is to the right of the 5, but usually not written, since there is no fractional or decimal portion to this number. The same number can be written as 645.0 or 645.00 or 645.000, etc. The position of the decimal place can change the entire value of a number, and impact a calculation. In the United States, the decimal place is used when representing money. You'll often be asked to round to a certain decimal place. Here is a review of some basic decimal **place value** names:

thousands	hundreds	tens	ones	tenths	hundredths	thousandths

↑ Decimal

The number 12,302.2 would be read as "twelve thousand, three hundred two and two-tenths."

In the United States, a period denotes the decimal place; however, some countries use a comma. The comma is used in the United States to separate thousands, millions, and so on.

To round to the nearest whole number (eliminating the decimal portion), the example would become 12,302. For rounding, go to the number that is one place to the right of what you are rounding to. If the number is 0 through 4, there will be no change. For numbers 5 through 9, round up to the next whole number.

Example: Round 6,423.7 to the ones place.

Since the tenths place is the position to the right of the ones place, we use that number to determine if we round up or not. In this case, the 3 is in the ones place and the 7 is in the tenths place. (6,423.7)

The 7 in the tenths place means we round the 3 up, so the final number will be 6,424.0

Example: Round 542.88 to the nearest tens

Since the ones place is the position to the right of the tens, we use that number to determine if we round up or not. In this case, the 4 is in the tens place and the 2 is in the ones place (542.88).

The 2 in the ones place means we do not round the 4 up, so the final number will be 540.00

Note: Everything to the right of the rounded position goes to 0 as a placeholder.

Example: Say you wanted to post an advertisement to sell a used vehicle for $2,000.00. However, when typing the price, you accidentally moved the decimal over one place to the left. Now the asking price appears as $200.00. This difference of a factor of 10 is dramatic. As numbers get bigger or smaller, the impact of this mistake becomes more pronounced. If you were looking to sell a condo for $1,000,000.00, but made an error and moved the decimal place to the left one position, the price posts at $100,000.00. A mistake of a factor of 10 cost $900,000.00.

In dividing by 10, you move the decimal one position to the left, making a smaller number than the original. If multiplying by 10, move the decimal one position to the right, making a larger number than the original.

Example: Divide 100 by 10 or $100 \div 10$.

Move the decimal one place to the left, so the result is a smaller number than the original.

$$100 \div 10 = 10$$

Example: Divide 1.0 by 10 or $1.0 \div 10$.

Move the decimal one place to the left, so the result is a smaller number than the original.

$$1.0 \div 10 = 0.1$$

Example: Multiply 100 by 10 or 100×10.

Move the decimal one place to the right, so the result is a larger number than the original.

$$100 \times 10 = 1{,}000$$

Example: Multiply 0.1 by 10 or 0.1×10.

Move the decimal one place to the right, so the result is a larger number than the original.

$$0.1 \times 10 = 1.0$$

Prefixes

Moving the decimal place to the left or to the right illustrates multiplying or dividing by factors of 10. The metric system of units for measurement utilizes factors of 10 as displayed in the following table:

kilo	1,000 units
hecto	100 units
deca	10 units
base unit	
deci	0.1 units
centi	0.01 units
milli	0.001 units

It is important to have the ability to quickly manipulate by 10 according to prefixes for units.

Example: How many milliliters are in 5 liters of saline solution?

There are 1,000 milliliters for every 1 liter. If we have 5 liters, it would be $5 \times 1{,}000 = 5{,}000 \text{ mL}$.

You may also count the zeros and which side of the decimal place they are on: 1,000 has three zeroes to the left of the decimal, so insert three zeroes between the 5 and the decimal, or move the decimal place over three places to the right, for your answer of 5,000 mL.

Example: How many kilograms are in 4.8 grams?

There is 1 gram for every 0.001 kilograms. Since there is one-thousandth of a kilogram for each gram, that means divide by 1,000, or move the decimal to the left by 3 places–1 place for each 0. So, the result would be 0.0048 kg.

For quick conversions, move the decimal place the set number of spaces left or right to match the column/slot, as depicted below.

To convert from one prefix to another to the left or right of the base unit (follow the arrow to the left or right), move the decimal place the number of columns/slots as counted.

mega			kilo	hecto	deca	base	deci	centi	milli			micro
1,000,000	100,000	10,000	1,000	100	10	unit	.1	.01	.001	.0001	.00001	.000001

← move decimal to the left | move decimal to the right →

Example: How many centiliters are in 4.7 kiloliters?

To convert a number with a unit prefixed as kilo into a unit prefixed as centi, move across five columns to the right, meaning move the decimal place five places to the right.

$$4.7 \text{ kL} = 470{,}000 \text{ cL}$$

Example: How many liters are in 30 microliters?

Start with the unit marked micro and count the columns moving to the left until you reach the base unit for liters. Be sure to count the blank columns, as they are important placeholders. There are six columns from micro to the base unit moving to the left, so move the decimal place six places to the left.

$$30 \text{ mL} = 0.000030 \text{ L}$$

Operations with Decimals

Addition

Addition with decimals is done the same way as regular addition. All numbers could have decimals, but are often removed if the numbers to the right of the decimal are zeros. Line up numbers at the decimal place.

Example: Add $345.89 + 23.54$

Line the numbers up at the decimal place and add.

$$\begin{array}{r} 345.89 \\ +\ 23.54 \\ \hline 369.43 \end{array}$$

Subtraction

Subtraction with decimals is done the same way as regular subtraction.

Example: Subtract $345.89 - 23.54$

Line the numbers up at the decimal place and subtract.

$$\begin{array}{r} 345.89 \\ -\ 23.54 \\ \hline 322.35 \end{array}$$

Multiplication

The simplest way to handle multiplication with decimals is to calculate the multiplication problem pretending the decimals are not there, then count how many decimal places there are in the original problem. Use that total to place the decimal the same number of places over, counting from right to left.

Example: Multiply 42.33×3.3

Line the numbers up and multiply, pretending there are no decimals.

$$\begin{array}{r} 4233 \\ \times\ \ 33 \\ \hline 12699 \\ 126990 \\ \hline 139689 \end{array}$$

Now look at the original problem and count how many decimal places were removed. Two decimal places were removed from 42.33 to get 4,233, and one decimal place from 3.3 to get 33. Removed were

$2 + 1 = 3$ decimal places. Place the decimal three places from the right of the number 139,689. The answer is 139.689.

Another way to think of this is that when you move the decimal in the original numbers, it is like multiplying by 10. To put the decimals back, you need to divide the number by 10 the same amount of times you multiplied. It would still be three times for the above solution.

Example: Multiply 0.03×1.22

Line the numbers up and multiply, pretending there are no decimals. The zeroes in front of the 3 are unnecessary, so take them out for now.

$$\begin{array}{r} 122 \\ \times \quad 3 \\ \hline 366 \end{array}$$

Look at the original problem and count how many decimals places were removed, or how many times each number was multiplied by 10. The 1.22 moved two places (or multiplied by 10 twice), as did 0.03. That is $2 + 2 = 4$ decimal places removed. Count that number, from right to left of the number 366, and place the decimal. The result is 0.0366.

Decimal Division

Division with decimals is simplest when you eliminate some of the decimal places. Since you divide the bottom number of a fraction into the top, or divide the denominator into the numerator, the bottom number dictates the movement of the decimals. The goal is to remove the decimals from the denominator and mirror that movement in the numerator. You do not need the numerator to be decimal free, however. Divide as you would normally.

Example:

Divide $4.21/0.2$ or $4.21 \div 0.2$

Move the decimal over one place to the right in the denominator, making 0.2 simply 2. Move the decimal in the numerator, 4.21, over the same amount, so it is now 42.1.

$$0.2\overline{)4.21}$$

Becomes

$$2\overline{)42.1}$$

Divide.

$$\begin{array}{r} 21.05 \\ 2\overline{)42.10} \end{array}$$

The answer is 21.05 with the correct decimal placement. In decimal division, move the decimal the same amount for both numerator and denominator. There is no need to adjust anything after the problem is completed.

Fractions

A **fraction** is an expression that represents a part of a whole but can also be used to present ratios or division problems. An example of a fraction is $\frac{x}{y}$. In this example, x is called the **numerator**, while y is the **denominator**. The numerator represents the number of parts, and the denominator is the total number of parts. They are separated by a line or slash, known as a **fraction bar**. In simple fractions, the numerator and denominator can be nearly any integer. However, the denominator of a fraction can never be zero because dividing by zero is a function that is undefined.

Imagine that an apple pie has been baked for a holiday party, and the full pie has eight slices. After the party, there are five slices left. How could the amount of the pie that remains be expressed as a fraction? The numerator is 5 since there are 5 pieces left, and the denominator is 8 since there were eight total slices in the whole pie. Thus, expressed as a fraction, the leftover pie totals $\frac{5}{8}$ of the original amount.

Fractions come in three different varieties: proper fractions, improper fractions, and mixed numbers. **Proper fractions** have a numerator less than the denominator, such as $\frac{3}{8}$, but **improper fractions** have a numerator greater than the denominator, such as $\frac{7}{2}$. **Mixed numbers** combine a whole number with a proper fraction, such as $3\frac{1}{2}$. Any mixed number can be written as an improper fraction by multiplying the integer by the denominator, adding the product to the value of the numerator, and dividing the sum by the original denominator. For example:

$$3\frac{1}{2} = \frac{3 \times 2 + 1}{2} = \frac{7}{2}$$

Whole numbers can also be converted into fractions by placing the whole number as the numerator and making the denominator 1. For example, $3 = \frac{3}{1}$.

One of the most fundamental concepts of fractions is their ability to be manipulated by multiplication or division. This is possible since $\frac{\mathrm{n}}{\mathrm{n}} = 1$ for any non-zero integer. As a result, multiplying or dividing by $\frac{\mathrm{n}}{\mathrm{n}}$ will not alter the original fraction since any number multiplied or divided by 1 doesn't change the value of that number. Fractions of the same value are known as equivalent fractions. For example, $\frac{2}{4}, \frac{4}{8}, \frac{50}{100}$, and $\frac{75}{150}$ are equivalent, as they all equal $\frac{1}{2}$.

Although many equivalent fractions exist, they are easier to compare and interpret when reduced or simplified. The numerator and denominator of a simple fraction will have no factors in common other than 1. When reducing or simplifying fractions, divide the numerator and denominator by the **greatest common factor**. A simple strategy is to divide the numerator and denominator by low numbers, like 2, 3, or 5 until arriving at a simple fraction, but the same thing could be achieved by determining the greatest common factor for both the numerator and denominator and dividing each by it. Using the first method is preferable when both the numerator and denominator are even, end in 5, or are obviously a multiple of another number. However, if no numbers seem to work, it will be necessary to factor the numerator and denominator to find the GCF. For example:

1) Simplify the fraction $\frac{6}{8}$:

Dividing the numerator and denominator by 2 results in $\frac{3}{4}$, which is a simple fraction.

2) Simplify the fraction $\frac{12}{36}$:

Dividing the numerator and denominator by 2 leaves $\frac{6}{18}$. This isn't a simple fraction, as both the numerator and denominator have factors in common. Dividing each by 3 results in $\frac{2}{6}$, but this can be further simplified by dividing by 2 to get $\frac{1}{3}$. This is the simplest fraction, as the numerator is 1. In cases like this, multiple division operations can be avoided by determining the greatest common factor between the numerator and denominator. The greatest common factor of $\frac{12}{36}$ is 12 because it divides evenly into both numbers, equaling $\frac{1}{3}$.

3) Simplify the fraction $\frac{18}{54}$ by dividing by the greatest common factor:

First, determine the factors for the numerator and denominator. The factors of 18 are 1, 2, 3, 6, 9, and 18. The factors of 54 are 1, 2, 3, 6, 9, 18, 27, and 54. Thus, the greatest common factor is 18. Dividing both the numerator and denominator by 18 leaves $\frac{1}{3}$, which is the simplest fraction. This method takes slightly more work, but it definitively arrives at the simplest fraction.

Operations with Fractions

Of the four basic operations that can be performed on fractions, the one that involves the least amount of work is multiplication. To multiply two fractions, simply multiply the numerators together, multiply the denominators together, and place the products of each as a fraction. Whole numbers and mixed numbers can also be expressed as a fraction, as described above, to multiply with a fraction. Here are a few examples:

1) $\frac{2}{5} \times \frac{3}{4} = \frac{6}{20} = \frac{3}{10}$

2) $\frac{4}{9} \times \frac{7}{11} = \frac{28}{99}$

Dividing fractions is similar to multiplication with one key difference. To divide fractions, flip the numerator and denominator of the second fraction, and then proceed as if it were a multiplication problem:

1) $\frac{7}{8} \div \frac{4}{5} = \frac{7}{8} \times \frac{5}{4} = \frac{35}{32}$

2) $\frac{5}{9} \div \frac{1}{3} = \frac{5}{9} \times \frac{3}{1} = \frac{15}{9} = \frac{5}{3}$

Addition and subtraction require more steps than multiplication and division, as these operations require the fractions to have the same denominator, also called a **common denominator**. It is always possible to find a common denominator by multiplying the denominators. However, when the denominators are large numbers, this method is unwieldy, especially if the answer must be provided in its simplest form. Thus, it's beneficial to find the **least common denominator** of the fractions—the least common denominator is incidentally also the least common multiple.

Once equivalent fractions have been found with common denominators, simply add or subtract the numerators to arrive at the answer:

1) $\frac{1}{2}+\frac{3}{4}=\frac{2}{4}+\frac{3}{4}=\frac{5}{4}$

2) $\frac{3}{12}+\frac{11}{20}=\frac{15}{60}+\frac{33}{60}=\frac{48}{60}=\frac{4}{5}$

3) $\frac{7}{9}-\frac{4}{15}=\frac{35}{45}-\frac{12}{45}=\frac{23}{45}$

4) $\frac{5}{6}-\frac{7}{18}=\frac{15}{18}-\frac{7}{18}=\frac{8}{18}=\frac{4}{9}$

Changing Fractions to Decimals

To change a fraction into a decimal, divide the denominator into the numerator until there are no remainders. There may be repeating decimals, so rounding is often acceptable. A straight line above the repeating portion denotes that the decimal repeats.

Example: Express $\frac{4}{5}$ as a decimal.

Set up the division problem.

$$5\overline{)4}$$

5 does not go into 4, so place the decimal and add a zero.

$$5\overline{)4.0}$$

5 goes into 40 eight times. There is no remainder.

$$\begin{array}{r} 0.8 \\ 5\overline{)4.0} \\ -\,4.0 \\ \hline 0 \end{array}$$

The solution is 0.8.

Example: Express $33\frac{1}{3}$ as a decimal.

Since the whole portion of the number is known, set it aside to calculate the decimal from the fraction portion.

Set up the division problem.

$$3\overline{)1}$$

3 does not go into 1, so place the decimal and add zeros. 3 goes into 10 three times.

$$\begin{array}{r} 0.3 \\ 3\overline{)1.0} \end{array}$$

This will repeat with a remainder of 1.

$$\begin{array}{r} 0.333 \\ 3\overline{)1.000} \\ -9 \\ \hline 10 \\ -9 \\ \hline 10 \end{array}$$

So, we will place a line over the 3 to denote the repetition. The solution is written $33.\overline{3}$.

Changing Decimals to Fractions

To change decimals to fractions, place the decimal portion of the number, the numerator, over the respective place value, the denominator, then reduce, if possible.

Example

Express 0.25 as a fraction.

This is read as twenty-five hundredths, so put 25 over 100. Then reduce to find the solution.

$$\frac{25}{100} = \frac{1}{4}$$

Example

Express 0.455 as a fraction.

This is read as four hundred fifty-five thousandths, so put 455 over 1,000. Then reduce to find the solution.

$$\frac{455}{1{,}000} = \frac{91}{200}$$

There are two types of problems that commonly involve percentages. The first is to calculate some percentage of a given quantity, where you convert the percentage to a decimal, and multiply the quantity by that decimal. Secondly, you are given a quantity and told it is a fixed percent of an unknown quantity. In this case, convert to a decimal, then divide the given quantity by that decimal.

Example

What is 30% of 760?

Convert the percent into a useable number. "Of" means to multiply.

$$30\% = 0.30$$

Set up the problem based on the givens and solve.

$$0.30 \times 760 = 228$$

Example

8.4 is 20% of what number?

Convert the percent into a useable number.

$$20\% = 0.20$$

The given number is a percent of the answer needed, so divide the given number by this decimal rather than multiplying it.

$$\frac{8.4}{0.20} = 42$$

Ratios and Proportions

Ratios

Ratios are used to show the relationship between two quantities. The ratio of oranges to apples in the grocery store may be 3 to 2. That means that for every 3 oranges, there are 2 apples. This comparison can be expanded to represent the actual number of oranges and apples, such as 36 oranges to 24 apples. Another example may be the number of boys to girls in a math class. If the ratio of boys to girls is given as 2 to 5, that means there are 2 boys to every 5 girls in the class. Ratios can also be compared if the units in each ratio are the same. The ratio of boys to girls in the math class can be compared to the ratio of boys to girls in a science class by stating which ratio is higher and which is lower.

Rates are used to compare two quantities with different units. Unit rates are the simplest form of rate. With **unit rates**, the denominator in the comparison of two units is one. For example, if someone can type at a rate of 1,000 words in 5 minutes, then their unit rate for typing is $\frac{1{,}000}{5} = 200$ words in one minute or 200 words per minute. Any rate can be converted into a unit rate by dividing to make the denominator one. 1,000 words in 5 minutes has been converted into the unit rate of 200 words per minute.

Ratios and rates can be used together to convert rates into different units. For example, if someone is driving 50 kilometers per hour, that rate can be converted into miles per hour by using a ratio known as the **conversion factor**. Since the given value contains kilometers and the final answer needs to be in miles, the ratio relating miles to kilometers needs to be used. There are 0.62 miles in 1 kilometer. This, written as a ratio and in fraction form, is $\frac{0.62 \text{ miles}}{1 \text{ km}}$. To convert 50km/hour into miles per hour, the following conversion needs to be set up:

$$\frac{50 \text{ km}}{\text{hour}} \times \frac{0.62 \text{ miles}}{1 \text{ km}} = 31 \text{ miles per hour}$$

The ratio between two similar geometric figures is called the **scale factor**. For example, a problem may depict two similar triangles, A and B. The scale factor from the smaller triangle A to the larger triangle B is given as 2 because the length of the corresponding side of the larger triangle, 16, is twice the corresponding side on the smaller triangle, 8. This scale factor can also be used to find the value of a missing side, x, in triangle A. Since the scale factor from the smaller triangle (A) to larger one (B) is 2, the larger corresponding side in triangle B (given as 25) can be divided by 2 to find the missing side in A ($x = 12.5$). The scale factor can also be represented in the equation $2A = B$ because two times the lengths of A gives the corresponding lengths of B. This is the idea behind similar triangles.

Proportions

Much like a scale factor can be written using an equation like $2A = B$, a **relationship** is represented by the equation $Y = kX$. X and Y are proportional because as values of X increase, the values of Y also increase. A relationship that is inversely proportional can be represented by the equation $Y = \frac{k}{X}$, where the value of Y decreases as the value of X increases and vice versa.

Proportional reasoning can be used to solve problems involving ratios, percentages, and averages. Ratios can be used in setting up proportions and solving them to find unknowns. For example, if a student completes an average of 10 pages of math homework in 3 nights, how long would it take the student to complete 22 pages? Both ratios can be written as fractions. The second ratio would contain the unknown.

The following proportion represents this problem, where x is the unknown number of nights:

$$\frac{10 \text{ pages}}{3 \text{ nights}} = \frac{22 \text{ pages}}{x \text{ nights}}$$

Solving this proportion entails cross-multiplying (multiplying both sets of numbers that are diagonally across and setting them equal to each other) and results in the following equation: $10x = 22 \times 3$. Simplifying and solving for x results in the exact solution: $x = 6.6 \text{ nights}$. The result would be rounded up to 7 because the homework would actually be completed on the 7th night.

The following problem uses ratios involving percentages:

If 20% of the class is girls and 30 students are in the class, how many girls are in the class?

To set up this problem, it is helpful to use the common proportion: $\frac{\%}{100} = \frac{is}{of}$. Within the proportion, % is the percentage of girls, 100 is the total percentage of the class, *is* is the number of girls, and *of* is the total number of students in the class. Most percentage problems can be written using this language. To solve this problem, the proportion should be set up as $\frac{20}{100} = \frac{x}{30}$, and then solved for x. Cross-multiplying results in the equation $20 \times 30 = 100x$, which results in the solution $x = 6$. There are 6 girls in the class.

Ratios can be used to solve problems that concern length, volume, and other units. For example, a problem may ask for the volume of a cone to be found that has a radius, $r = 7$ m and a height, $h = 16$ m. Referring to the formulas provided on the test, the volume of a cone is given as: $V = \pi r^2 \frac{h}{3}$, where r is the radius, and h is the height. Plugging $r = 7$ and $h = 16$ into the formula, the following is obtained:

$$V = \pi(7^2)\frac{16}{3}$$

Therefore, the volume of the cone is found to be approximately 821 m^3. Sometimes, answers in different units are sought. If this problem wanted the answer in liters, 821 m^3 would need to be converted. Using the equivalence statement $1 \text{ m}^3 = 1{,}000 \text{ L}$, the following ratio would be used to solve for liters:

$$821\text{m}^3 \times \frac{1{,}000 \text{ L}}{1 \text{ m}^3}$$

Cubic meters in the numerator and denominator cancel each other out, and the answer is converted to 821,000 liters, or 8.21×10^5 L.

Other conversions can also be made between different given and final units. If the temperature in a pool is 30°C, what is the temperature of the pool in degrees Fahrenheit? To convert these units, an equation is used relating Celsius to Fahrenheit. The following equation is used:

$$T_{°F} = 1.8T_{°C} + 32$$

Plugging in the given temperature and solving the equation for T yields the result:

$$T_{°F} = 1.8(30) + 32 = 86°F$$

Units in both the metric system and U.S. customary system are widely used.

Here are some more examples of how to solve for proportions:

1) $\frac{75\%}{90\%} = \frac{25\%}{x}$

To solve for x, the fractions must be cross multiplied:

$$75\%x = 90\% \times 25\%$$

To make things easier, let's convert the percentages to decimals:

$$0.9 \times 0.25 = 0.225 = 0.75x$$

To get rid of x's coefficient, each side must be divided by that same coefficient to get the answer $x = 0.3$. The question could ask for the answer as a percentage or fraction in lowest terms, which are 30% and $\frac{3}{10}$, respectively.

2) $\frac{x}{12} = \frac{30}{96}$

Cross-multiply: $96x = 30 \times 12$
Multiply: $96x = 360$
Divide: $x = 360 \div 96$
Answer: $x = 3.75$

3) $\frac{0.5}{3} = \frac{x}{6}$

Cross-multiply: $3x = 0.5 \times 6$
Multiply: $3x = 3$
Divide: $x = 3 \div 3$
Answer: $x = 1$

You may have noticed there's a faster way to arrive at the answer. If there is an obvious operation being performed on the proportion, the same operation can be used on the other side of the proportion to solve for x. For example, in the first practice problem, 75% became 25% when divided by 3, and upon doing the same to 90%, the correct answer of 30% would have been found with much less legwork. However, these questions aren't always so intuitive, so it's a good idea to work through the steps, even if the answer seems apparent from the outset.

Percentages

Think of percentages as fractions with a denominator of 100. In fact, **percentage** means "per hundred." Problems often require converting numbers from percentages, fractions, and decimals. The following explains how to work through those conversions.

Conversions

Decimals and Percentages: Since a percentage is based on "per hundred," decimals and percentages can be converted by multiplying or dividing by 100. Practically speaking, this always amounts to moving the decimal point two places to the right or left, depending on the conversion. To convert a percentage to a decimal, move the decimal point two places to the left and remove the % sign. To convert a decimal to a percentage, move the decimal point two places to the right and add a % sign.

Here are some examples:

$65\% = 0.65$
$0.33 = 33\%$
$0.215 = 21.5\%$
$99.99\% = 0.9999$
$500\% = 5.00$

$$7.55 = 755\%$$

Fractions and Percentages: Remember that a percentage is a number per one hundred. So, a percentage can be converted to a fraction by making the number in the percentage the numerator and putting 100 as the denominator:

$$43\% = \frac{43}{100}$$

$$97\% = \frac{97}{100}$$

$$4.7\% = \frac{47}{1{,}000}$$

Note in the last example, that the decimal can be removed by going from 100 to 1,000, because it's accomplished by multiplying the numerator and denominator by 10.

Note that the percent symbol (%) kind of looks like a 0, a 1, and another 0. So, think of a percentage like 54% as 54 over 100. Note that it's often good to simplify a fraction into the smallest possible numbers. So, $\frac{54}{100}$ would then become 27/50:

$$\frac{54}{100} \div \frac{2}{2} = \frac{27}{50}$$

To convert a fraction to a percent, follow the same logic. If the fraction happens to have 100 in the denominator, you're in luck. Just take the numerator and add a percent symbol:

$$\frac{28}{100} = 28\%$$

Another option is to make the denominator equal to 100. Be sure to multiply the numerator and the denominator by the same number. For example:

$$\frac{3}{20} \times \frac{5}{5} = \frac{15}{100}$$

$$\frac{15}{100} = 15\%$$

If neither of those strategies work, divide the numerator by the denominator to get a decimal:

$$\frac{9}{12} = 0.75$$

Then convert the decimal to a percentage:

$$0.75 = 75\%$$

Percent Formula

The percent formula looks like this:

$$\frac{part}{whole} = \frac{\%}{100}$$

After numbers are plugged in, multiply the diagonal numbers and then divide by the remaining one. It works every time.

So, when a question asks what percent 5 is of 10, plug the numbers in like this:

$$\frac{5}{10} = \frac{\%}{100}$$

Multiply the diagonal numbers:

$$5 \times 100 = 500$$

Divide by the remaining number:

$$\frac{500}{10} = 50\%$$

The percent formula can be applied in a number of different circumstances by plugging in the numbers appropriately.

Exponents

An **exponent** is an operation used as shorthand for a number multiplied or divided by itself for a defined number of times:

$$3^7 = 3 \times 3 \times 3 \times 3 \times 3 \times 3 \times 3$$

In this example, the 3 is called the base, and the 7 is called the exponent. The exponent is typically expressed as a superscript number near the upper-right side of the base but can also be identified as the number following a caret symbol (^). This operation would be verbally expressed as "3 to the 7th power" or "3 raised to the power of 7." Common exponents are 2 and 3. A base raised to the power of 2 is referred to as having been "squared," while a base raised to the power of 3 is referred to as having been "cubed."

Several special rules apply to exponents. First, the Zero Power Rule finds that any number raised to the zero power equals 1. For example, 100^0, 2^0, $(-3)^0$and 0^0 all equal 1 because the bases are raised to the zero power.

Second, exponents can be negative. With negative exponents, the equation is expressed as a fraction, as in the following example:

$$3^{-7} = \frac{1}{3^7} = \frac{1}{3 \times 3 \times 3 \times 3 \times 3 \times 3 \times 3}$$

Third, the Power Rule concerns exponents being raised by another exponent. When this occurs, the exponents are multiplied by each other:

$$(x^2)^3 = x^6 = (x^3)^2$$

Fourth, when multiplying two exponents with the same base, the Product Rule requires that the base remains the same, and the exponents are added. For example, $a^x \times a^y = a^{x+y}$. Since addition and multiplication are commutative, the two terms being multiplied can be in any order.

$$x^3x^5 = x^{3+5} = x^8 = x^{5+3} = x^5x^3$$

Fifth, when dividing two exponents with the same base, the Quotient Rule requires that the base remains the same, but the exponents are subtracted. So, $a^x \div a^y = a^{x-y}$. Since subtraction and division are not commutative, the two terms must remain in order.

$$x^5x^{-3} = x^{5-3} = x^2 = x^5 \div x^3 = \frac{x^5}{x^3}$$

Additionally, 1 raised to any power is still equal to 1, and any number raised to the power of 1 is equal to itself. In other words, $a^1 = a$ and $14^1 = 14$.

Exponents play an important role in scientific notation to present extremely large or small numbers as follows: $a \times 10^b$. To write the number in scientific notation, the decimal is moved until there is only one digit on the left side of the decimal point, indicating that the number a has a value between 1 and 10. The number of times the decimal moves indicates the exponent to which 10 is raised, here represented by b. If the decimal moves to the left, then b is positive, but if the decimal moves to the right, then b is negative.

See the following examples:

$$3{,}050 = 3.05 \times 10^3$$

$$-777 = -7.77 \times 10^2$$

$$0.000123 = 1.23 \times 10^{-4}$$

$$-0.0525 = -5.25 \times 10^{-2}$$

Roots

The **square root symbol** is expressed as $\sqrt{\ }$ and is commonly known as the radical. Taking the root of a number is the inverse operation of multiplying that number by itself some amount of times. For example, squaring the number 7 is equal to 7×7, or 49. Finding the square root is the opposite of finding an exponent, as the operation seeks a number that when multiplied by itself equals the number in the square root symbol.

For example, $\sqrt{36} = 6$ because 6 multiplied by 6 equals 36. Note, the square root of 36 is also -6 since $-6 \times -6 = 36$. This can be indicated using a plus/minus symbol like this: ± 6. However, square roots are often just expressed as a positive number for simplicity with it being understood that the true value can be either positive or negative.

Perfect squares are square roots that are whole numbers. The list of perfect squares begins with 0, 1, 4, 9, 16, 25, 36, 49, 64, 81, and 100.

Determining the square root of imperfect squares requires a calculator to reach an exact figure. It's possible, however, to approximate the answer by finding the two perfect squares that the number fits between. For example, the square root of 40 is between 6 and 7 since the squares of those numbers are 36 and 49, respectively.

Square roots are the most common root operation. If the radical doesn't have a number to the upper left of the symbol $\sqrt{}$, then it's a square root. Sometimes a radical includes a number in the upper left, like $\sqrt[3]{27}$, as in the other common root type—the cube root. Complicated roots like the cube root often require a calculator.

Parentheses

Parentheses separate different parts of an equation, and operations within them should be thought of as taking place before the outside operations take place. Practically, this means that the distinction between what is inside and outside of the parentheses decides the order of operations that the equation follows. Failing to solve operations inside the parentheses before addressing the part of the equation outside of the parentheses will lead to incorrect results.

For example, let's analyze $5 - (3 + 25)$. The addition operation within the parentheses must be solved first. So $3 + 25 = 28$, leaving $5 - (28) = -23$. If this was solved in the incorrect order of operations, the solution might be found to be $5 - 3 + 25 = 2 + 25 = 27$, which would be wrong.

Equations often feature multiple layers of parentheses. To differentiate them, square brackets [ ] and braces { } are used in addition to parentheses. The innermost parentheses must be solved before working outward to larger brackets. For example, in $\{2 \div [5 - (3 + 1)]\}$, solving the innermost parentheses $(3 + 1)$ leaves $\{2 \div [5 - (4)]\}$. $[5 - (4)]$ is now the next smallest, which leaves $\{2 \div [1]\}$ in the final step, and 2 as the answer.

Order of Operations

When solving equations with multiple operations, special rules apply. These rules are known as the **Order of Operations**. The order is as follows: Parentheses, Exponents, Multiplication and Division from left to right, and Addition and Subtraction from left to right. A popular pneumonic device to help remember the order is Please Excuse My Dear Aunt Sally (PEMDAS).

Evaluate the following two problems to understand the Order of Operations:

1) $4 + (3 \times 2)^2 \div 4$

First, solve the operation within the parentheses: $4 + 6^2 \div 4$.
Second, solve the exponent: $4 + 36 \div 4$.
Third, solve the division operation: $4 + 9$.
Fourth, finish the operation with addition for the answer, 13.

2) $2 \times (6 + 3) \div (2 + 1)^2$

$2 \times 9 \div (3)^2$
$2 \times 9 \div 9$
$18 \div 9$
2

Comparing and Ordering Rational Numbers

A common question type asks test takers to order rational numbers from least to greatest or greatest to least. The numbers will come in a variety of formats, including decimals, percentages, roots, fractions, and whole numbers. These questions test for knowledge of different types of numbers and the ability to determine their respective values.

Whether the question asks to order the numbers from greatest to least or least to greatest, the crux of the question is the same—convert the numbers into a common format. Generally, it's easiest to write the numbers as whole numbers and decimals so they can be placed on a number line.

Follow these examples to understand this strategy.

1) Order the following rational numbers from greatest to least:

$$\sqrt{36}, 0.65, 78\%, \frac{3}{4}, 7, 90\%, \frac{5}{2}$$

Of the seven numbers, the whole number (7) and decimal (0.65) are already in an accessible form, so concentrate on the other five.

First, the square root of 36 equals 6. (If the test asks for the root of a non-perfect root, determine which two whole numbers the root lies between.) Next, convert the percentages to decimals. A percentage means "per hundred," so this conversion requires moving the decimal point two places to the left, leaving 0.78 and 0.9. Lastly, evaluate the fractions:

$$\frac{3}{4} = \frac{75}{100} = 0.75\,; \frac{5}{2} = 2\frac{1}{2} = 2.5$$

Now, the only step left is to list the numbers in the requested order:

$$7, \sqrt{36}, \frac{5}{2}, 90\%, 78\%, \frac{3}{4}, 0.65$$

2) Order the following rational numbers from least to greatest:

$$2.5, \sqrt{9}, -10.5, 0.853, 175\%, \sqrt{4}, \frac{4}{5}$$

$$\sqrt{9} = 3$$

$$175\% = 1.75$$

$$\sqrt{4} = 2$$

$$\frac{4}{5} = 0.8$$

From least to greatest, the answer is:

$$-10.5, \frac{4}{5}, 0.853, 175\%, \sqrt{4}, 2.5, \sqrt{9}$$

Word Problems

Translating Verbal Relationships into Algebraic Equations or Expressions

When attempting to solve a math problem, it's important to apply the correct algorithm. It is much more difficult to determine what algorithm is necessary when solving word problems, because the necessary operations and equations are typically not provided. In these instances, the test taker must translate the words in the problem into true mathematical statements that can be solved. The following are examples:

Symbol	Phrase
+	Added to; increased by; sum of; more than
−	Decreased by; difference between; less than; take away
×	Multiplied by; 3(4,5...) times as large; product of
÷	Divided by; quotient of; half (third, etc.) of
=	Is; the same as; results in; as much as; equal to
x, t, n, etc.	A number; unknown quantity; value of; variable

Addition and subtraction are **inverse operations**. Adding a number and then subtracting the same number will cancel each other out, resulting in the original number, and vice versa. For example, $8 + 7 - 7 = 8$ and $137 - 100 + 100 = 137$. Similarly, multiplication and division are inverse operations. Therefore, multiplying by a number and then dividing by the same number results in the original number, and vice versa. For example, $8 \times 2 \div 2 = 8$ and $12 \div 4 \times 4 = 12$. Inverse operations are used to work backwards to solve problems. In the case that 7 and a number add to 18, the inverse operation of subtraction is used to find the unknown value $(18 - 7 = 11)$. If a school's entire 4th grade was divided evenly into 3 classes each with 22 students, the inverse operation of multiplication is used to determine the total students in the grade $(22 \times 3 = 66)$. Additional scenarios involving inverse operations are included in the tables below.

There are a variety of real-world situations in which one or more of the operators is used to solve a problem. The tables below display the most common scenarios.

Addition & Subtraction

	Unknown Result	Unknown Change	Unknown Start
Adding to	5 students were in class. 4 more students arrived. How many students are in class? $5 + 4 = ?$	8 students were in class. More students arrived late. There are now 18 students in class. How many students arrived late? $8 + ? = 18$ Solved by inverse operations $18 - 8 = ?$	Some students were in class early. 11 more students arrived. There are now 17 students in class. How many students were in class early? $? + 11 = 17$ Solved by inverse operations $17 - 11 = ?$
Taking from	15 students were in class. 5 students left class. How many students are in class now? $15 - 5 = ?$	12 students were in class. Some students left class. There are now 8 students in class. How many students left class? $12 - ? = 8$ Solved by inverse operations $8 + ? = 12 \rightarrow 12 - 8 = ?$	Some students were in class. 3 students left class. Then there were 13 students in class. How many students were in class before? $? - 3 = 13$ Solved by inverse operations $13 + 3 = ?$

	Unknown Total	Unknown Addends (Both)	Unknown Addends (One)
Putting together/ taking apart	The homework assignment is 10 addition problems and 8 subtraction problems. How many problems are in the homework assignment? $10 + 8 = ?$	Bobby has $9. How much can Bobby spend on candy and how much can Bobby spend on toys? $9 = ? + ?$	Bobby has 12 pairs of pants. 5 pairs of pants are shorts, and the rest are long. How many pairs of long pants does he have? $12 = 5 + ?$ Solved by inverse operations $12 - 5 = ?$

	Unknown Difference	Unknown Larger Value	Unknown Smaller Value
Comparing	Bobby has 5 toys. Tommy has 8 toys. How many more toys does Tommy have than Bobby? $5 + ? = 8$ Solved by inverse operations $8 - 5 = ?$ Bobby has \$6. Tommy has \$10. How many fewer dollars does Bobby have than Tommy? $10 - 6 = ?$	Tommy has 2 more toys than Bobby. Bobby has 4 toys. How many toys does Tommy have? $2 + 4 = ?$ Bobby has 3 fewer dollars than Tommy. Bobby has \$8. How many dollars does Tommy have? $? - 3 = 8$ Solved by inverse operations $8 + 3 = ?$	Tommy has 6 more toys than Bobby. Tommy has 10 toys. How many toys does Bobby have? $? + 6 = 10$ Solved by inverse operations $10 - 6 = ?$ Bobby has \$5 less than Tommy. Tommy has \$9. How many dollars does Bobby have? $9 - 5 = ?$

Multiplication and Division

	Unknown Product	Unknown Group Size	Unknown Number of Groups
Equal groups	There are 5 students, and each student has 4 pieces of candy. How many pieces of candy are there in all? $5 \times 4 = ?$	14 pieces of candy are shared equally by 7 students. How many pieces of candy does each student have? $7 \times ? = 14$ Solved by inverse operations $14 \div 7 = ?$	If 18 pieces of candy are to be given out 3 to each student, how many students will get candy? $? \times 3 = 18$ Solved by inverse operations $18 \div 3 = ?$

	Unknown Product	Unknown Factor	Unknown Factor
Arrays	There are 5 rows of students with 3 students in each row. How many students are there? $5 \times 3 = ?$	If 16 students are arranged into 4 equal rows, how many students will be in each row? $4 \times ? = 16$ Solved by inverse operations $16 \div 4 = ?$	If 24 students are arranged into an array with 6 columns, how many rows are there? $? \times 6 = 24$ Solved by inverse operations $24 \div 6 = ?$

	Larger Unknown	Smaller Unknown	Multiplier Unknown
Comparing	A small popcorn costs \$1.50. A large popcorn costs 3 times as much as a small popcorn. How much does a large popcorn cost? $1.50 \times 3 = ?$	A large soda costs \$6 and that is 2 times as much as a small soda costs. How much does a small soda cost? $2 \times ? = 6$ Solved by inverse operations $6 \div 2 =?$	A large pretzel costs \$3 and a small pretzel costs \$2. How many times as much does the large pretzel cost as the small pretzel? $? \times 2 = 3$ Solved by inverse operations $3 \div 2 = ?$

Modeling and Solving Word Problems

Some word problems require more than just one simple equation to be written and solved. Consider the following situations and the linear equations used to model them.

Suppose Margaret is 2 miles to the east of John at noon. Margaret walks to the east at 3 miles per hour. How far apart will they be at 3 p.m.? To solve this, x would represent the time in hours past noon, and y would represent the distance between Margaret and John. Now, noon corresponds to the equation where x is 0, so the y-intercept is going to be 2. It's also known that the slope will be the rate at which the distance is changing, which is 3 miles per hour.

This means that the slope will be 3 (be careful at this point: if units were used, other than miles and hours, for x and y variables, a conversion of the given information to the appropriate units would be required first). The simplest way to write an equation given the y-intercept, and the slope is the Slope-Intercept form, which is $y = mx + b$. Recall that m here is the slope and b is the y-intercept. So, $m = 3$ and $b = 2$. Therefore, the equation will be $y = 3x + 2$. The word problem asks how far to the east Margaret will be from John at 3 p.m., which means when x is 3. So, substitute $x = 3$ into this equation to obtain:

$$y = 3 \times 3 + 2 = 9 + 2 = 11$$

Therefore, she will be 11 miles to the east of him at 3 p.m.

For another example, suppose that a box with 4 cans in it weighs 6 lbs., while a box with 8 cans in it weighs 12 lbs. Find out how much a single can weighs. To do this, let x denote the number of cans in the box, and y denote the weight of the box with the cans in lbs. This line touches two pairs: $(4, 6)$ and (8, 12). A formula for this relation could be written using the two-point form, with $x_1 = 4, y_1 = 6, x_2 = 8, y_2 = 12$. This would yield $\frac{y-6}{x-4} = \frac{12-6}{8-4}$, or $\frac{y-6}{x-4} = \frac{6}{4} = \frac{3}{2}$. However, only the slope is needed to solve this problem, since the slope will be the weight of a single can. From the computation, the slope is $\frac{3}{2}$. Therefore, each can weighs $\frac{3}{2}$ lb.

Working with Money

Walter's Coffee Shop sells a variety of drinks and breakfast treats.

Price List	
Hot Coffee	$2.00
Slow-Drip Iced Coffee	$3.00
Latte	$4.00
Muffin	$2.00
Crepe	$4.00
Egg Sandwich	$5.00

Costs	
Hot Coffee	$0.25
Slow-Drip Iced Coffee	$0.75
Latte	$1.00
Muffin	$1.00
Crepe	$2.00
Egg Sandwich	$3.00

Walter's utilities, rent, and labor costs him $500 per day. Today, Walter sold 200 hot coffees, 100 slow-drip iced coffees, 50 lattes, 75 muffins, 45 crepes, and 60 egg sandwiches. What was Walter's total profit today?

To accurately answer this type of question, determine the total cost of making his drinks and treats, then determine how much revenue he earned from selling those products. After arriving at these two totals, the profit is measured by deducting the total cost from the total revenue.

Walter's costs for today:

Item	Quantity	Cost Per Unit	Total Cost
Hot Coffee	200	$0.25	$50
Slow-Drip Iced Coffee	100	$0.75	$75
Latte	50	$1.00	$50
Muffin	75	$1.00	$75
Crepe	45	$2.00	$90
Egg Sandwich	60	$3.00	$180
Utilities, rent, and labor			$500
Total Costs			$1,020

Walter's revenue for today:

Item	Quantity	Revenue Per Unit	Total Revenue
Hot Coffee	200	$2.00	$400
Slow-Drip Iced Coffee	100	$3.00	$300
Latte	50	$4.00	$200
Muffin	75	$2.00	$150
Crepe	45	$4.00	$180
Egg Sandwich	60	$5.00	$300
Total Revenue			$1,530

This strategy is applicable to other question types. For example, calculating salary after deductions, balancing a checkbook, and calculating a dinner bill are common word problems similar to business planning. Just remember to use the correct operations. When a balance is increased, use addition. When a balance is decreased, use subtraction. Common sense and organization are your greatest assets when answering word problems.

Solving Real-World Problems Involving Percentages

Questions dealing with percentages can be difficult when they are phrased as word problems. These word problems almost always come in three varieties. The first type will ask to find what percentage of some number will equal another number. The second asks to determine what number is some percentage of another given number. The third will ask what number another number is a given percentage of.

One of the most important parts of correctly answering percentage word problems is to identify the numerator and the denominator. This fraction can then be converted into a percentage, as described above.

The following word problem shows how to make this conversion:

> A department store carries several different types of footwear. The store is currently selling 8 athletic shoes, 7 dress shoes, and 5 sandals. What percentage of the store's footwear are sandals?

First, calculate what serves as the "whole," as this will be the denominator. How many total pieces of footwear does the store sell? The store sells 20 different types (8 athletic + 7 dress + 5 sandals).

Second, what footwear type is the question specifically asking about? Sandals. Thus, 5 is the numerator.

Third, the resultant fraction must be expressed as a percentage. The first two steps indicate that $\frac{5}{20}$ of the footwear pieces are sandals. This fraction must now be converted into a percentage:

$$\frac{5}{20} \times \frac{5}{5} = \frac{25}{100} = 25\%$$

Solving Real-World Problems Involving Proportions

Much like a scale factor can be written using an equation like $2A = B$, a relationship is represented by the equation $Y = kX$. X and Y are proportional because as values of X increase, the values of Y also increase. A relationship that is inversely proportional can be represented by the equation $Y = \frac{k}{X}$, where the value of Y decreases as the value of x increases and vice versa.

Proportional reasoning can be used to solve problems involving ratios, percentages, and averages. Ratios can be used in setting up proportions and solving them to find unknowns. For example, if a student completes an average of 10 pages of math homework in 3 nights, how long would it take the student to complete 22 pages? Both ratios can be written as fractions. The second ratio would contain the unknown.

The following proportion represents this problem, where x is the unknown number of nights:

$$\frac{10 \text{ pages}}{3 \text{ nights}} = \frac{22 \text{ pages}}{x \text{ nights}}$$

Solving this proportion entails cross-multiplying and results in the following equation:

$$10x = 22 \times 3$$

Simplifying and solving for x results in the exact solution: $x = 6.6$ nights. The result would be rounded up to 7 because the homework would actually be completed on the 7th night.

The following problem uses ratios involving percentages:

> If 20% of the class is girls and 30 students are in the class, how many girls are in the class?

To set up this problem, it is helpful to use the common proportion:

$$\frac{\%}{100} = \frac{is}{of}$$

Within the proportion, % is the percentage of girls, 100 is the total percentage of the class, *is* is the number of girls, and *of* is the total number of students in the class. Most percentage problems can be written using this language. To solve this problem, the proportion should be set up as $\frac{20}{100} = \frac{x}{30}$, and then solved for x. Cross-multiplying results in the equation $20 \times 30 = 100x$, which results in the solution $x = 6$. There are 6 girls in the class.

Problems involving volume, length, and other units can also be solved using ratios. For example, a problem may ask for the volume of a cone to be found that has a radius, $r = 7\text{ m}$ and a height, $h = 16\text{ m}$. Referring to the formulas provided on the test, the volume of a cone is given as: $V = \pi r^2 \frac{h}{3}$, where r is the radius, and h is the height. Plugging $r = 7$ and $h = 16$ into the formula, the following is obtained:

$$V = \pi(7^2)\frac{16}{3}$$

Therefore, the volume of the cone is found to be approximately 821m^3. Sometimes, answers in different units are sought. If this problem wanted the answer in liters, 821m^3 would need to be converted. Using the equivalence statement $1\text{ m}^3 = 1{,}000\text{ L}$, the following ratio would be used to solve for liters:

$$821\text{m}^3 \times \frac{1{,}000\text{ L}}{1\text{ m}^3}$$

Cubic meters in the numerator and denominator cancel each other out, and the answer is converted to 821,000 liters, or $8.21 \times 10^5\text{ L}$.

Other conversions can also be made between different given and final units. If the temperature in a pool is 30°C, what is the temperature of the pool in degrees Fahrenheit? To convert these units, an equation is used relating Celsius to Fahrenheit. The following equation is used:

$$T_{°F} = 1.8T_{°C} + 32$$

Plugging in the given temperature and solving the equation for T yields the result:

$$T_{°F} = 1.8(30) + 32 = 86°\text{F}$$

Units in both the metric system and U.S. customary system are widely used.

Here are some more examples of how to solve for proportions:

1) $\frac{75\%}{90\%} = \frac{25\%}{x}$

To solve for x, the fractions must be cross multiplied: $75\%x = 90\% \times 25\%$. To make things easier, let's convert the percentages to decimals: $0.9 \times 0.25 = 0.225 = 0.75x$. To get rid of x's coefficient, each side must be divided by that same coefficient to get the answer $x = 0.3$. The question could ask for the answer as a percentage or fraction in lowest terms, which are 30% and $\frac{3}{10}$, respectively.

2) $\frac{x}{12} = \frac{30}{96}$

Cross-multiply: $96x = 30 \times 12$
Multiply: $96x = 360$
Divide: $x = 360 \div 96$
Answer: $x = 3.75$

3) $\frac{0.5}{3} = \frac{x}{6}$

Cross-multiply: $3x = 0.5 \times 6$
Multiply: $3x = 3$
Divide: $x = 3 \div 3$
Answer: $x = 1$

You may have noticed there's a faster way to arrive at the answer. If there is an obvious operation being performed on the proportion, the same operation can be used on the other side of the proportion to solve for x. For example, in the first practice problem, 75% became 25% when divided by 3, and upon doing the same to 90%, the correct answer of 30% would have been found with much less legwork. However, these questions aren't always so intuitive, so it's a good idea to work through the steps, even if the answer seems apparent from the outset.

Solving Real-World Problems Involving Unit Rate

Unit rate word problems will ask to calculate the rate or quantity of something in a different value. For example, a problem might say that a car drove a certain number of miles in a certain number of minutes and then ask how many miles per hour the car was traveling. These questions involve solving proportions. Consider the following examples:

1) Alexandra made $96 during the first 3 hours of her shift as a temporary worker at a law office. She will continue to earn money at this rate until she finishes in 5 more hours. How much does Alexandra make per hour? How much will Alexandra have made at the end of the day?

This problem can be solved in two ways. The first is to set up a proportion, as the rate of pay is constant. The second is to determine her hourly rate, multiply the 5 hours by that rate, and then add the $96.

To set up a proportion, put the money already earned over the hours already worked on one side of an equation. The other side has x over 8 hours (the total hours worked in the day). It looks like this: $\frac{96}{3} = \frac{x}{8}$. Now, cross-multiply to get $768 = 3x$. To get x, divide by 3, which leaves $x = 256$. Alternatively, as *x* is the numerator of one of the proportions, multiplying by its denominator will reduce the solution by one step. Thus, Alexandra will make $256 at the end of the day. To calculate her hourly rate, divide the total by 8, giving $32 per hour.

Alternatively, it is possible to figure out the hourly rate by dividing $96 by 3 hours to get $32 per hour. Now her total pay can be figured by multiplying $32 per hour by 8 hours, which comes out to $256.

2) Jonathan is reading a novel. So far, he has read 215 of the 335 total pages. It takes Jonathan 25 minutes to read 10 pages, and the rate is constant. How long does it take Jonathan to read one page? How much longer will it take him to finish the novel? Express the answer in time.

To calculate how long it takes Jonathan to read one page, divide the 25 minutes by 10 pages to determine the page per minute rate. Thus, it takes 2.5 minutes to read one page.

Jonathan must read 120 more pages to complete the novel. (This is calculated by subtracting the pages already read from the total.) Now, multiply his rate per page by the number of pages. Thus, $120 \times 2.5 = 300$. Expressed in time, 300 minutes is equal to 5 hours.

3) At a hotel, $\frac{4}{5}$ of the 120 rooms are booked for Saturday. On Sunday, $\frac{3}{4}$ of the rooms are booked. On which day are more of the rooms booked, and by how many more?

The first step is to calculate the number of rooms booked for each day. Do this by multiplying the fraction of the rooms booked by the total number of rooms.

Saturday: $\frac{4}{5} \times 120 = \frac{4}{5} \times \frac{120}{1} = \frac{480}{5} = 96 \text{ rooms}$

Sunday: $\frac{3}{4} \times 120 = \frac{3}{4} \times \frac{120}{1} = \frac{360}{4} = 90 \text{ rooms}$

Thus, more rooms were booked on Saturday by 6 rooms.

4) In a veterinary hospital, the veterinarian-to-pet ratio is 1:9. The ratio is always constant. If there are 45 pets in the hospital, how many veterinarians are currently in the veterinary hospital?

Set up a proportion to solve for the number of veterinarians: $\frac{1}{9} = \frac{x}{45}$

Cross-multiplying results in $9x = 45$, which works out to 5 veterinarians.

Alternatively, as there are always 9 times as many pets as veterinarians, it is possible to divide the number of pets (45) by 9. This also arrives at the correct answer of 5 veterinarians.

5) At a general practice law firm, 30% of the lawyers work solely on tort cases. If 9 lawyers work solely on tort cases, how many lawyers work at the firm?

First, solve for the total number of lawyers working at the firm, which will be represented here with x. The problem states that 9 lawyers work solely on torts cases, and they make up 30% of the total lawyers at the firm. Thus, 30% multiplied by the total, x, will equal 9. Written as equation, this is: $30\% \times x = 9$.

It's easier to deal with the equation after converting the percentage to a decimal, leaving $0.3x = 9$. Thus, $x = \frac{9}{0.3} = 30$ lawyers working at the firm.

6) Xavier was hospitalized with pneumonia. He was originally given 35mg of antibiotics. Later, after his condition continued to worsen, Xavier's dosage was increased to 60mg. What was the percent increase of the antibiotics? Round the percentage to the

An increase or decrease in percentage can be calculated by dividing the difference in amounts by the original amount and multiplying by 100. Written as an equation, the formula is:

$$\frac{new\ quantity - old\ quantity}{old\ quantity} \times 100$$

Here, the question states that the dosage was increased from 35mg to 60mg, so these are plugged into the formula to find the percentage increase.

$$\frac{60 - 35}{35} \times 100 = \frac{25}{35} \times 100$$

$$0.7142 \times 100 = 71.4\%$$

Solving Simple Algebraic Problems

Linear equations and **linear inequalities** are both comparisons of two algebraic expressions. However, unlike equations in which the expressions are equal, linear inequalities compare expressions that may be unequal. Linear equations typically have one value for the variable that makes the statement true. Linear inequalities generally have an infinite number of values that make the statement true.

When solving a linear equation, the desired result requires determining a numerical value for the unknown variable. If given a linear equation involving addition, subtraction, multiplication, or division, working backwards isolates the variable. Addition and subtraction are inverse operations, as are multiplication and division. Therefore, they can be used to cancel each other out.

Since variables are the letters that represent an unknown number, you must solve for that unknown number in single variable problems. The main thing to remember is that you can do anything to one side of an equation as long as you do it to the other.

The first steps to solving linear equations are distributing, if necessary, and combining any like terms on the same side of the equation. Sides of an equation are separated by an equal sign. Next, the equation is manipulated to show the variable on one side. Again, whatever is done to one side of the equation must be done to the other side of the equation to remain equal. Inverse operations are then used to isolate the variable and undo the order of operations backwards. Addition and subtraction are undone, then multiplication and division are undone.

> For example, solve $4(t - 2) + 2t - 4 = 2(9 - 2t)$
>
> Distributing: $4t - 8 + 2t - 4 = 18 - 4t$
>
> Combining like terms: $6t - 12 = 18 - 4t$
>
> Adding $4t$ to each side to move the variable: $10t - 12 = 18$
>
> Adding 12 to each side to isolate the variable: $10t = 30$
>
> Dividing each side by 10 to isolate the variable: $t = 3$

The answer can be checked by substituting the value for the variable into the original equation and ensuring that both sides calculate to be equal.

Converting Within and Between Standard and Metric Systems

American Measuring System

The measuring system used today in the United States developed from the British units of measurement during colonial times. The most typically used units in this customary system are those used to measure weight, liquid volume, and length, whose common units are found below. In the customary system, the basic unit for measuring weight is the ounce (oz); there are 16 ounces (oz) in 1 pound (lb) and 2,000 pounds in 1 ton. The basic unit for measuring liquid volume is the ounce (oz); 1 ounce is equal to 2 tablespoons (tbsp) or 6 teaspoons (tsp), and there are 8 ounces in 1 cup, 2 cups in 1 pint (pt), 2 pints in 1 quart (qt), and 4 quarts in 1 gallon (gal). For measurements of length, the inch (in) is the base unit; 12 inches make up 1 foot (ft), 3 feet make up 1 yard (yd), and 5,280 feet make up 1 mile (mi).

However, as there are only a set number of units in the customary system, with extremely large or extremely small amounts of material, the numbers can become awkward and difficult to compare. Here is a conversion chart for common customary measurements:

Common Customary Measurements		
Length	**Weight**	**Capacity**
$1 \text{ foot} = 12 \text{ inches}$	$1 \text{ pound} = 16 \text{ ounces}$	$1 \text{ cup} = 8 \text{ fluid ounces}$
$1 \text{ yard} = 3 \text{ feet}$	$1 \text{ ton} = 2{,}000 \text{ pounds}$	$1 \text{ pint} = 2 \text{ cups}$
$1 \text{ yard} = 36 \text{ inches}$		$1 \text{ quart} = 2 \text{ pints}$
$1 \text{ mile} = 1{,}760 \text{ yards}$		$1 \text{ quart} = 4 \text{ cups}$
$1 \text{ mile} = 5{,}280 \text{ feet}$		$1 \text{ gallon} = 4 \text{ quarts}$
		$1 \text{ gallon} = 16 \text{ cups}$

Metric System

Aside from the United States, most countries in the world have adopted the **metric system** embodied in the International System of Units (SI). The three main SI base units used in the metric system are the meter (m), the kilogram (kg), and the liter (L); meters measure length, kilograms measure mass, and liters measure volume.

These three units can use different prefixes, which indicate larger or smaller versions of the unit by powers of ten. This can be thought of as making a new unit, which is sized by multiplying the original unit in size by a factor.

These prefixes and associated factors are:

Metric Prefixes			
Prefix	**Symbol**	**Multiplier**	**Exponential**
kilo	k	1,000	10^3
hecto	h	100	10^2
deca	da	10	10^1
no prefix		1	10^0
deci	d	0.1	10^{-1}
centi	c	0.01	10^{-2}
milli	m	0.001	10^{-3}

The correct prefix is then attached to the base. Some examples:

1 milliliter equals .001 liters.

1 kilogram equals 1,000 grams.

Choosing the Appropriate Measuring Unit

Some units of measure are represented as square or cubic units depending on the solution. For example, perimeter is measured in linear units (e.g., 24 in), area is measured in square units (e.g., 4 in^2) and volume is measured in cubic units (e.g., 50 cm^3).

Also be sure to use the most appropriate unit for the thing being measured. A building's height might be measured in feet or meters while the length of a nail might be measured in inches or centimeters. Additionally, for SI units, the prefix should be chosen to provide the most succinct available value. For example, the mass of a bag of fruit would likely be measured in kilograms rather than grams or milligrams, and the length of a bacteria cell would likely be measured in micrometers rather than centimeters or kilometers.

Conversion

Converting measurements in different units between the two systems can be difficult because they follow different rules. The best method is to look up an English to Metric system conversion factor and then use a series of equivalent fractions to set up an equation to convert the units of one of the measurements into those of the other.

The table below lists some common conversion values that are useful for problems involving measurements with units in both systems:

English System	Metric System
1 inch	2.54 cm
1 foot	0.3048 m
1 yard	0.914 m
1 mile	1.609 km
1 ounce	28.35 g
1 pound	0.454 kg
1 fluid ounce	29.574 mL
1 quart	0.946 L
1 gallon	3.785 L

Consider the example where a scientist wants to convert 6.8 inches to centimeters. The table above is used to find that there are 2.54 centimeters in every inch, so the following equation should be set up and solved:

$$\frac{6.8 \text{ in}}{1} \times \frac{2.54 \text{ cm}}{1 \text{ in}} = 17.272 \text{ cm}$$

Notice how the inches in the numerator of the initial figure and the denominator of the conversion factor cancel out. (This equation could have been written simply as $6.8 \text{ in} \times 2.54 \text{ cm} = 17.272 \text{ cm}$, but it was shown in detail to illustrate the steps). The goal in any conversion equation is to set up the fractions so that the units you are trying to convert from cancel out and the units you desire remain.

For a more complicated example, consider converting 2.15 kilograms into ounces. The first step is to convert kilograms into grams and then grams into ounces. Note that the measurement you begin with does not have to be put in a fraction.

So, in this case, 2.15 kg is by itself although it's technically the numerator of a fraction:

$$2.15\text{ kg} \times \frac{1{,}000\text{g}}{\text{kg}} = 2{,}150\text{ g}$$

Then, use the conversion factor from the table to convert grams to ounces:

$$2{,}150\text{ g} \times \frac{1\text{ oz}}{28.35\text{ g}} = 75.8\text{ oz}$$

Practice Quiz

1. A bucket can hold 11.4 liters of water. A kiddie pool needs 35 gallons of water to be full. How many times will the bucket need to be filled to fill the kiddie pool? (Use the conversion 1 gallon = 3.8 liters.)
   a. 12
   b. 35
   c. 11
   d. 45

2. In Jim's school, there are a total of 650 students. There are three girls for every two boys. How many students are girls?
   a. 260 girls
   b. 130 girls
   c. 65 girls
   d. 390 girls

3. Convert 0.351 to a percentage.
   a. 3.51%
   b. 35.1%
   c. $\frac{351}{100}$
   d. 0.00351%

4. Convert $\frac{2}{9}$ to a percentage.
   a. 22.22%
   b. 4.5%
   c. 450%
   d. 0.22%

5. Convert 57% to a decimal.
   a. 570
   b. 5.70
   c. 0.06
   d. 0.57

See answers on the next page.

Answer Explanations

1. A: Calculate how many gallons the bucket holds.

$$11.4 \text{ L} \times \frac{1 \text{ gal}}{3.8 \text{ L}} = 3 \text{ gal}$$

Next, calculate how many buckets are needed to fill the 35-gallon pool.

$$\frac{35}{3} = 11.67$$

Since the amount is more than 11 but less than 12, the bucket must be filled 12 times.

$3:2$**2. D:** Three girls for every two boys can be expressed as a ratio, . This can be visualized as splitting the school into 5 groups: 3 girl groups and 2 boy groups. The number of students in each group can be found by dividing the total number of students by 5:

$$\frac{650 \text{ students}}{5 \text{ groups}} = \frac{130 \text{ students}}{\text{group}}$$

To find the total number of girls, multiply the number of students per group (130) by the number of girl groups in the school (3). This equals 390, Choice *D.*

3. B: 35.1%

To convert from a decimal to a percentage, the decimal needs to be moved two places to the right. In this case, that makes 0.351 become 35.1%.

4. A: Converting a fraction to a percentage takes two steps. First, divide the numerator by the denominator to turn the fraction into a decimal:

$$\frac{2}{9} = 0.2222 \ldots$$

The "..." indicates a repeating decimal with an infinite number of 2's.

Now, to convert to a percentage, move the decimal point two places to the right:

$$22.22\%$$

5. D: 0.57

To convert from a percentage to a decimal, or vice versa, you always need to move the decimal two places. A percentage like 57% has an invisible decimal after the 7, like this:

$$57.\%$$

That decimal point needs to be moved two places to the left to get:

$$0.57$$

Science

General Terminology

Anatomy may be defined as the structural makeup of an organism. The study of anatomy may be divided into microscopic/fine anatomy and macroscopic/gross anatomy. **Fine anatomy** concerns itself with viewing the features of the body with the aid of a microscope, while **gross anatomy** concerns itself with viewing the features of the body with the naked eye. **Physiology** refers to the functions of an organism, and it examines the chemical or physical functions that help the body function appropriately.

Levels of Organization of the Human Body

All the parts of the human body are built of individual units called **cells**. Groups of similar cells are arranged into **tissues**, different tissues are arranged into **organs**, and organs working together form entire **organ systems**. The human body has twelve organ systems that govern circulation, digestion, immunity, hormones, movement, support, coordination, urination & excretion, reproduction (male and female), respiration, and general protection.

Body Cavities

The body is partitioned into different hollow spaces that house organs. The human body contains the following cavities:

- **Cranial cavity**: The cranial cavity is surrounded by the skull and contains organs such as the brain and pituitary gland.
- **Thoracic cavity**: The thoracic cavity is encircled by the sternum (breastbone) and ribs. It contains organs such as the lungs, heart, trachea (windpipe), esophagus, and bronchial tubes.
- **Abdominal cavity**: The abdominal cavity is separated from the thoracic cavity by the diaphragm. It contains organs such as the stomach, gallbladder, liver, small intestines, and large intestines. The abdominal organs are held in place by a membrane called the peritoneum.
- **Pelvic cavity**: The pelvic cavity is enclosed by the pelvis, or bones of the hip. It contains organs such as the urinary bladder, urethra, ureters, anus, and rectum. It contains the reproductive organs as well. In females, the pelvic cavity also contains the uterus.
- **Spinal cavity**: The spinal cavity is surrounded by the vertebral column. The vertebral column has five regions: cervical, thoracic, lumbar, sacral, and coccygeal. The spinal cord runs through the middle of the spinal cavity.

Three Primary Body Planes

A **plane** is an imaginary flat surface. The three primary planes of the human body are frontal, sagittal, and transverse. The frontal, or coronal, plane is a vertical plane that or organ into front (anterior) and back (posterior) portions. The **sagittal plane** is a vertical plane that divides the body or organ into right and left sides. The **transverse plane** is a horizontal plane that divides the body or organ into upper and lower portions. In medical imaging, computed tomography (CT) scans are oriented only in the transverse plane; while magnetic resonance imaging (MRI) scans may be oriented in any of the three planes.

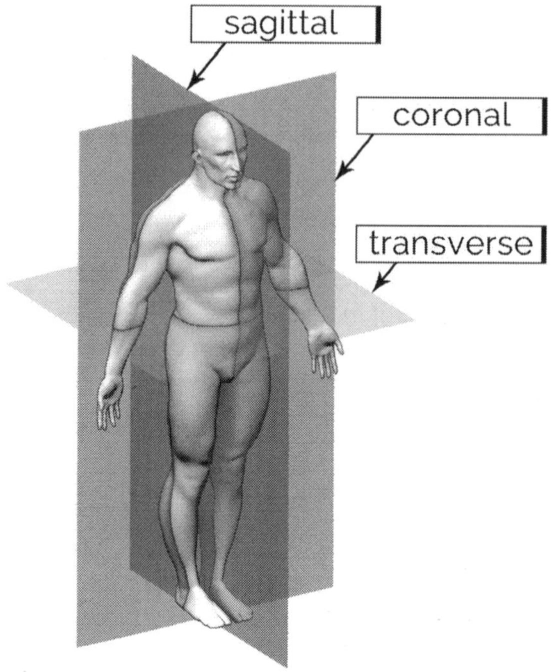

Note the body above is in the **anatomic position**. In anatomic position, the body and head are straight up and down, the feet are close but not touching, and the hands are pointed forward.

Terms of Direction

Medial refers to a structure being closer to the midline of the body. For example, the nose is medial to the eyes.

Lateral refers to a structure being farther from the midline of the body, and it is the opposite of medial. For example, the eyes are lateral to the nose.

Proximal refers to a structure or body part located near an attachment point. For example, the elbow is proximal to the wrist.

Distal refers to a structure or body part located far from an attachment point, and it is the opposite of proximal. For example, the wrist is distal to the elbow.

Anterior means toward the front in humans. For example, the lips are anterior to the teeth. The term ventral can be used in place of anterior and refers to the abdominal region, or underside, of an organism.

Posterior means toward the back in humans, and it is the opposite of anterior. For example, the teeth are posterior to the lips. The term dorsal can be used in place of posterior and refers to the back or upper side of an organism.

Superior means above and refers to a structure closer to the head. For example, the head is superior to the neck. The terms **cephalic** or **cranial** may be used in place of superior.

Inferior means below and refers to a structure farther from the head, and it is the opposite of superior. For example, the neck is inferior to the head. The term caudal may be used in place of inferior and refers to a structure near the tail or posterior of the body.

Superficial refers to a structure closer to the surface. For example, the muscles are superficial because they are just beneath the surface of the skin.

Deep refers to a structure farther from the surface, and it is the opposite of superficial. For example, the femur is a deep structure lying beneath the muscles.

Body Regions

Terms for general locations on the body include:

- Cervical: relating to the neck (can also refer to the cervix, as in cervical cancer)
- Clavicular: relating to the clavicle, or collarbone
- Ocular: relating to the eyes
- Acromial: relating to the shoulder
- Cubital: relating to the elbow
- Brachial: relating to the arm
- Carpal: relating to the wrist
- Thoracic: relating to the chest
- Abdominal: relating to the abdomen
- Pubic: relating to the groin
- Pelvic: relating to the pelvis, or bones of the hip
- Femoral: relating to the femur, or thigh bone
- Geniculate: relating to the knee
- Pedal: relating to the foot
- Palmar: relating to the palm of the hand
- Plantar: relating to the sole of the foot

Abdominopelvic Regions and Quadrants

The **abdominopelvic region** may be defined as the combination of the abdominal and the pelvic cavities. The region's upper border is the breasts and its lower border is the groin region. The region is divided into the following nine sections:

- Right hypochondriac: region below the cartilage of the ribs
- Epigastric: region above the stomach between the hypochondriac regions
- Left hypochondriac: region below the cartilage of the ribs
- Right lumbar: region of the waist
- Umbilical: region between the lumbar regions where the umbilicus, or belly button (navel), is located
- Left lumbar: region of the waist
- Right inguinal: region of the groin

- Hypogastric: region below the stomach between the inguinal regions
- Left inguinal: region of the groin

A simpler way to describe the abdominopelvic area is to divide it into the following quadrants:

- Right upper quadrant (RUQ): Encompasses the right hypochondriac, right lumbar, epigastric, and umbilical regions.
- Right lower quadrant (RLQ): Encompasses the right lumbar, right inguinal, hypogastric, and umbilical regions.
- Left upper quadrant (LUQ): Encompasses the left hypochondriac, left lumbar, epigastric, and umbilical regions.
- Left lower quadrant (LLQ): Encompasses the left lumbar, left inguinal, hypogastric, and umbilical regions.

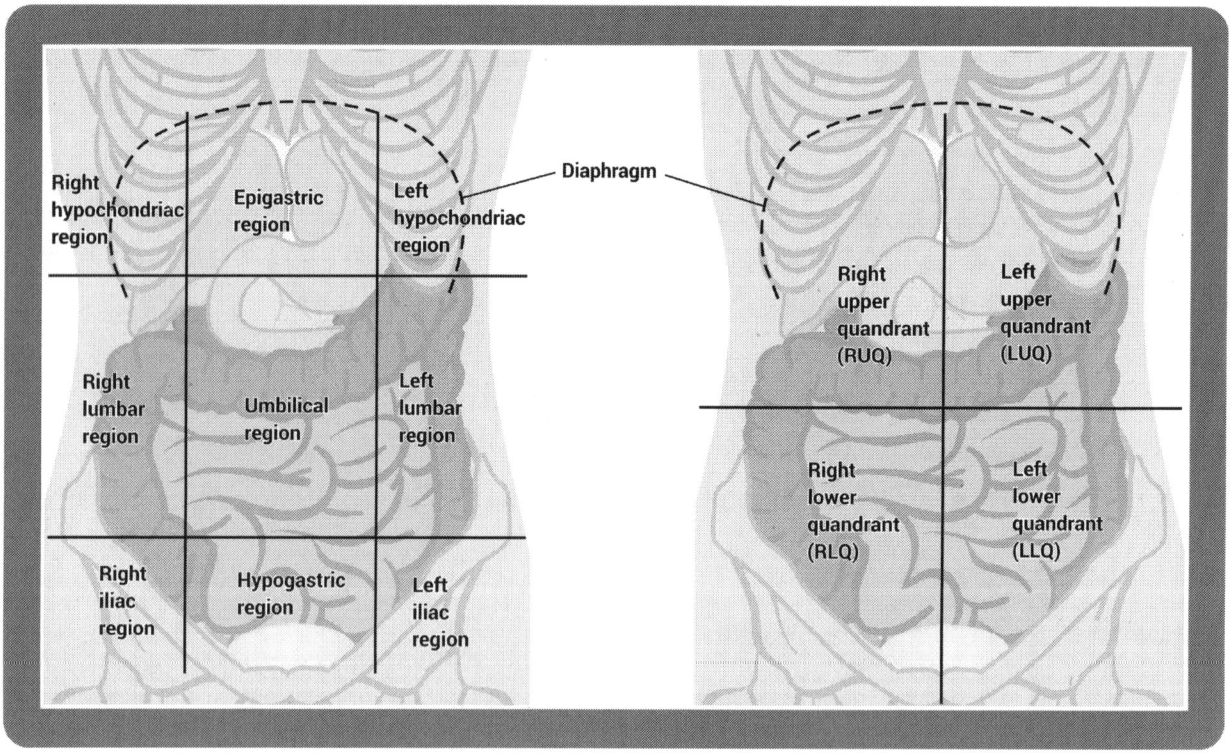

Histology

Histology is the examination of specialized cells and cell groups that perform a specific function by working together. Although there are trillions of cells in the human body, there are only 200 different types of cells. Groups of cells form biological tissues, and tissues combine to form organs, such as the heart and kidney. Organs are structures that have many different functions that are vital to living creatures. There are four primary types of tissue: epithelial, connective, muscle, and neural. Each tissue type has specific characteristics that enable organs and organ systems to function properly.

Muscle tissue supports the body and allows it to move, and muscles are special because their cells have the ability to contract. There are three distinct types of muscle tissue: skeletal, smooth, and cardiac. **Skeletal muscle** is voluntary, or under conscious control, and is usually attached to bones. Most body movement is directly caused by the contraction of skeletal muscle. **Smooth muscle** is typically involuntary, or not under conscious control, and may be found in blood vessels, the walls of hollow organs, and the urinary bladder. **Cardiac muscle** is involuntary and found in the heart, which helps propel blood throughout the body.

Nervous tissue is unique in that it is able to coordinate information from sensory organs as well as communicate the proper behavioral responses. **Neurons**, or nerve cells, are the workhorses of the nervous system. They communicate via **action potentials** (electrical signals) and **neurotransmitters** (chemical signals).

Epithelial tissue covers the external surfaces of organs and lines many of the body's cavities. Epithelial tissue helps to protect the body from invasion by microbes (bacteria, viruses, parasites), fluid loss, and injury.

Epithelial cell shapes can be:

- Squamous: cells with a flat shape
- Cuboidal: cells with a cubed shape
- Columnar: cells shaped like a column

Epithelial cells can be arranged in four patterns:

- Simple: a type of epithelium composed solely from a single layer of cells
- Stratified: a type of epithelium composed of multiple layers of cells
- Pseudostratified: a type of epithelium which appears to be stratified but, in reality, consists of only one layer of cells
- Transitional: a type of epithelium noted for its ability to expand and contract

Connective tissue supports and connects the tissues and organs of the body. Connective tissue is composed of cells dispersed throughout a matrix which can be gel, liquid, protein fibers, or salts. The primary protein fibers in the matrix are collagen (for strength), elastin (for flexibility), and reticulum (for support). Connective tissue can be categorized as either loose or dense. Examples of connective tissue include bones, cartilage, ligaments, tendons, blood, and adipose (fat) tissue.

Cardiovascular System

The **cardiovascular system** is a network of organs and tubes that transport blood, hormones, nutrients, oxygen, and other gases to cells and tissues throughout the body. It is also known as the cardiovascular system. The major components of the circulatory system are the blood vessels, blood, and heart. Blood will be discussed in the section on the hematological system.

Blood Vessels

In the circulatory system, **blood vessels** are responsible for transporting blood throughout the body. The three major types of blood vessels in the circulatory system are arteries, veins, and capillaries. **Arteries** carry blood from the heart to the rest of the body. Veins carry blood from the body back to the heart.

Capillaries connect arteries to veins and form networks that exchange materials between the blood and the cells.

In general, arteries are stronger and thicker than veins, as they withstand high pressures exerted by the blood as the heart pumps it through the body. Arteries control blood flow through either **vasoconstriction** (narrowing of the blood vessel's diameter) or **vasodilation** (widening of the blood vessel's diameter). The smallest arteries, which are farthest from the heart, are called **arterioles**. The blood in veins is under much lower pressures, so veins have valves to prevent the backflow of blood.

Most of the exchange between the blood and tissues takes place through the capillaries. There are three types of capillaries: continuous, fenestrated, and sinusoidal.

Continuous capillaries are made up of epithelial cells tightly connected together. As a result, they limit the types of materials that pass into and out of the blood. Continuous capillaries are the most common type of capillary. **Fenestrated capillaries** have openings that allow materials to be freely exchanged between the blood and tissues. They are commonly found in the digestive, endocrine, and urinary systems. **Sinusoidal capillaries** have larger openings and allow proteins and blood cells through. They are found primarily in the liver, bone marrow, and spleen.

Heart

The **heart** is a two-part, muscular pump that forcefully pushes blood throughout the human body. The human heart has four chambers—two upper atria and two lower ventricles separated by a partition called the septum. There is a pair on the left and a pair on the right. Anatomically, *left* and *right* correspond to the sides of the body that the patient themselves would refer to as left and right.

Four valves help to section off the chambers from one another. Between the right atrium and ventricle, the three flaps of the **tricuspid valve** keep blood from backflowing from the ventricle to the atrium, similar to how the two flaps of the **mitral valve** work between the left atrium and ventricle. As these two valves lie between an atrium and a ventricle, they are referred to as **atrioventricular (AV) valves**. The other two valves are **semilunar (SL)** and control blood flow into the two great arteries leaving the ventricles. The pulmonary valve connects the right ventricle to the pulmonary artery, while the aortic valve connects the left ventricle to the aorta.

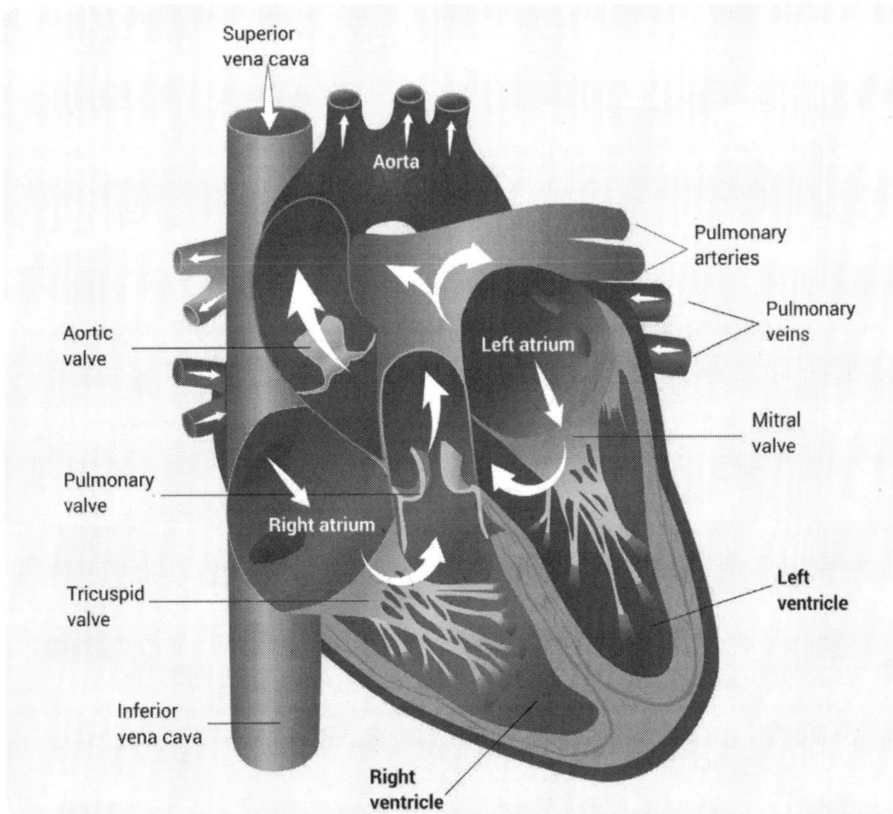

Cardiac Cycle

A **cardiac cycle** is one complete sequence of cardiac activity. The cardiac cycle represents the relaxation and contraction of the heart and can be divided into two phases: diastole and systole.

Diastole is the phase during which the heart relaxes and fills with blood. It gives rise to the diastolic blood pressure (DBP), which is the bottom number of a blood pressure reading. **Systole** is the phase during which the heart contracts and discharges blood. It gives rise to the systolic blood pressure (SBP), which is the top number of a blood pressure reading. The heart's electrical conduction system coordinates the cardiac cycle.

Types of Circulation

Five major blood vessels manage blood flow to and from the heart: the superior and inferior venae cavae, the aorta, the pulmonary artery, and the pulmonary vein.

The superior vena cava is a large vein that drains blood from the head and the upper body. The **inferior vena cava** is a large vein that drains blood from the lower body. The **aorta** is the largest artery in the human body and carries blood from the heart to body tissues. The **pulmonary arteries** carry blood from the heart to the lungs. The **pulmonary veins** transport blood from the lungs to the heart.

In the human body, there are two types of circulation: pulmonary circulation and systemic circulation. **Pulmonary circulation** supplies blood to the lungs. Deoxygenated blood enters the right atrium of the heart and is routed through the tricuspid valve into the right ventricle. Deoxygenated blood then travels from the right ventricle of the heart through the pulmonary valve and into the pulmonary arteries. The pulmonary arteries carry the deoxygenated blood to the lungs. In the lungs, oxygen is absorbed, and carbon dioxide is released. The pulmonary veins carry oxygenated blood to the left atrium of the heart.

Systemic circulation supplies blood to all other parts of the body, except the lungs. Oxygenated blood flows from the left atrium of the heart through the mitral, or bicuspid, valve into the left ventricle of the heart. Oxygenated blood is then routed from the left ventricle of the heart through the aortic valve and into the aorta. The aorta delivers blood to the systemic arteries, which supply the body tissues. In the tissues, oxygen and nutrients are exchanged for carbon dioxide and other wastes. The deoxygenated blood along with carbon dioxide and wastes enter the systemic veins, where they are returned to the right atrium of the heart via the superior and inferior vena cava.

Electrolytes

The five major electrolytes that are important to health are sodium, potassium, chloride, calcium, and magnesium. Sodium and potassium help to regulate the body's water balance and also play a significant role in muscle contraction. Chloride also helps with fluid balance and nerve conductions. Iron plays an important role in the body's ability to transport and use oxygen, and calcium is critical for bone formation, nerve conduction, and muscle contraction. Phosphorus is involved in intramuscular oxidation processes, and magnesium helps support energy metabolism.

Sweating can lower electrolytes and minerals such as sodium, potassium, chloride, iron, calcium, phosphorus, and magnesium. Electrolytes (sodium, potassium, and chloride) and water need to be replaced during extended exercise, particularly in hot and humid environments, because they are lost in sweat.

Sodium, which is needed to help maintain fluid balance, nerve function, muscle contractions, and acid-base balance, is the primary electrolyte lost in sweat and must be replaced. It is important to include sodium in fluids or food as part of the rehydration process, particularly after exercise, so that overhydration, or hyponatremia, does not occur as a result of drinking water alone. Adding sodium to fluids also helps to improve the absorption of water and carbohydrates. Most commercial sports drinks are formulated to provide the optimal levels of sodium and carbohydrates in solution.

Gastrointestinal System

The human body relies completely on the **gastrointestinal** or **digestive system** to meet its nutritional needs. After food and drink are ingested, the digestive system breaks them down into their component nutrients and absorbs them so that the circulatory system can transport them to other cells to use for growth, energy, and cell repair. These nutrients may be classified as proteins, lipids, carbohydrates, vitamins, and minerals.

The digestive system is thought of chiefly in two parts: the **digestive tract** and the accessory digestive organs. The digestive tract is the pathway in which food is ingested, digested, absorbed, and excreted. It is composed of the mouth, pharynx, esophagus, stomach, small and large intestines, rectum, and anus. **Peristalsis**, or wave-like contractions of smooth muscle, moves food and wastes through the digestive tract. The accessory digestive organs are the salivary glands, liver, gallbladder, and pancreas.

Mouth and Stomach

The **mouth** is the entrance to the digestive system. Here, the mechanical and chemical digestion of the food begins. The food is chewed mechanically by the teeth and shaped into a bolus by the tongue so that it can be more easily swallowed by the esophagus. The food also becomes waterier and more pliable with the addition of saliva secreted from the salivary glands, the largest of which are the parotid glands. The glands also secrete **amylase** in the saliva, an enzyme which begins chemical digestion and breakdown of the carbohydrates and sugars in the food.

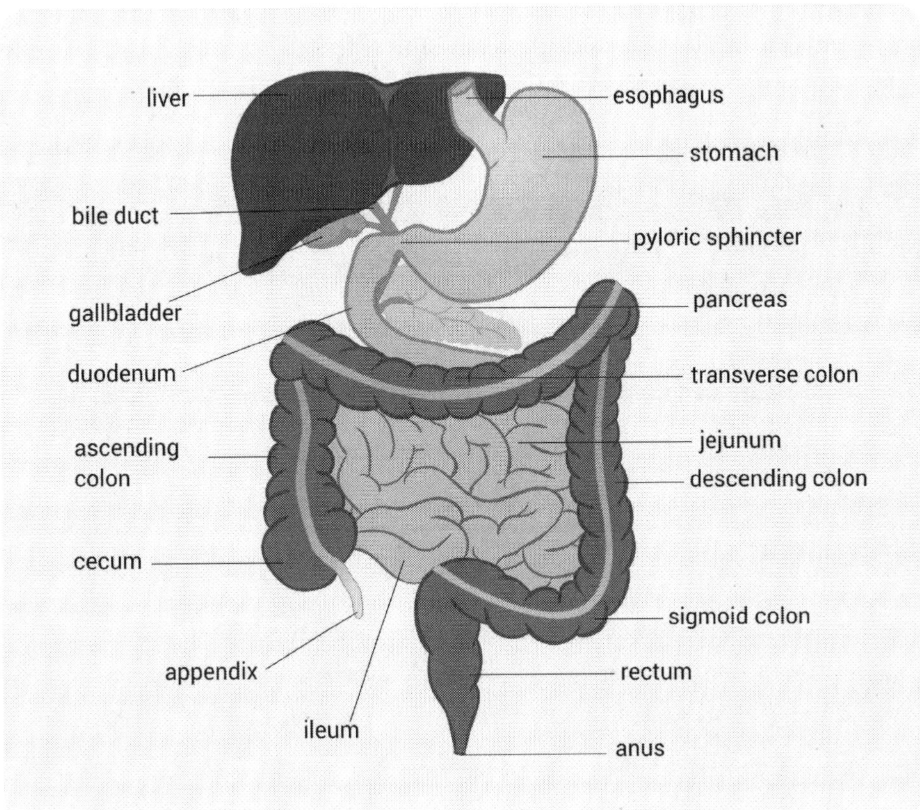

The food then moves through the pharynx and down the muscular esophagus to the stomach.

The **stomach** is a large, muscular sac-like organ at the distal end of the esophagus. Here, the bolus is subjected to more mechanical and chemical digestion. As it passes through the stomach, it is physically squeezed and crushed while additional secretions turn it into a watery nutrient-filled liquid that exits into the small intestine as **chyme**.

The stomach secretes a great many substances into the lumen of the digestive tract. Some cells produce gastrin, a hormone that prompts other cells in the stomach to secrete a gastric acid composed mostly of hydrochloric acid (HCl). The HCl is at such a high concentration and low pH that it denatures most proteins and degrades a lot of organic matter. The stomach also secretes mucous to form a protective film that keeps the corrosive acid from dissolving its own cells. Gaps in this mucous layer can lead to peptic ulcers. Finally, the stomach also uses digestive enzymes like proteases and lipases to break down proteins and fats; although there are some gastric lipases here, the stomach is most known for breaking down proteins.

Small Intestine

The chyme from the stomach enters the first part of the **small intestine**, the **duodenum**, through the pyloric sphincter, and its extreme acidity is partly neutralized by sodium bicarbonate secreted along with mucous. The presence of chyme in the duodenum triggers the secretion of the hormones secretin and cholecystokinin (CCK). Secretin acts on the pancreas to dump more sodium bicarbonate into the small intestine so that the pH is kept at a reasonable level, while CCK acts on the gallbladder to release the bile that it has been storing. Bile, a substance produced by the liver and stored in the gallbladder, helps to emulsify or dissolve fats and lipids.

Because of the bile (which aids in lipid absorption) and the secreted lipases (which break down fats), the duodenum is the chief site of fat digestion in the body. The duodenum also represents the last major site of chemical digestion in the digestive tract, as the other two sections of the small intestine (the jejunum and ileum) are instead heavily involved in absorption of nutrients.

The small intestine reaches forty feet in length, and its cells are arranged in small finger-like projections called **villi**. This is due to its key role in the absorption of nearly all nutrients from the ingested and digested food, effectively transferring them from the lumen of the GI tract to the bloodstream, where they travel to the cells that need them. These nutrients include simple sugars like glucose from carbohydrates, amino acids from proteins, emulsified fats, electrolytes like sodium and potassium, minerals like iron and zinc, and vitamins like D and B12. Vitamin B12's absorption, though it takes place in the intestines, is actually aided by **intrinsic factor** that was released into the chyme back in the stomach.

Large Intestine

The leftover parts of food which remain unabsorbed or undigested in the lumen of the small intestine next travel through the **large intestine**. The large intestine is mainly responsible for water absorption. As the chyme at this stage no longer has anything useful that can be absorbed by the body, it is now referred to as **waste**, and it is stored in the large intestine until it can be excreted from the body. Removing the liquid from the waste transforms it from liquid to solid stool, or **feces**.

This waste first passes from the small intestine to the cecum, a pouch that forms the first part of the large intestine. In herbivores, it provides a place for bacteria to digest cellulose, but in humans most of it is vestigial and is known as the **appendix**. From the cecum, waste next travels up the ascending colon, across the transverse colon, down the descending colon, and through the sigmoid colon to the rectum. The rectum is responsible for the final storage of waste before it is expelled through the anus. The anal canal is a small portion of the rectum leading through to the anus and the outside of the body.

Pancreas

The **pancreas** has endocrine and exocrine functions. The endocrine function involves releasing the hormone insulin, which decreases blood sugar (glucose) levels, and glucagon, which increases blood sugar (glucose) levels, directly into the bloodstream. Both hormones are produced in the **islets of Langerhans**, insulin in the beta cells and glucagon in the alpha cells.

The exocrine function of the pancreas involves the secretion of inactive digestive enzymes (zymogens) from acinar cells into the main pancreatic duct. The main pancreatic duct joins the common bile duct, which empties into the small intestine (specifically the duodenum). The digestive enzymes are then activated and take part in the digestion of carbohydrates, proteins, and fats within chyme (the mixture of partially digested food and digestive juices).

Immune System

The **immune system** is the body's defense against invading microorganisms (bacteria, viruses, fungi, and parasites) and other harmful, foreign substances. It is capable of limiting or preventing infection.

There are two general types of immunity: innate immunity and acquired immunity. **Innate immunity** uses physical and chemical barriers to block microorganism entry into the body. The biggest barrier is the skin; it forms a physical barrier that blocks microorganisms from entering underlying tissues. Mucous membranes in the digestive, respiratory, and urinary systems secrete mucus to block and remove invading microorganisms. Other natural defenses include saliva, tears, and stomach acids, which are all chemical barriers intended to block infection with microorganisms. Acid is inhospitable to pathogens, as are tears, mucus, and saliva, which all contain a natural antibiotic called lysozyme. The respiratory passages contain microscopic cilia, which are like bristles that sweep out pathogens. In addition, macrophages and other white blood cells can recognize and eliminate foreign objects through phagocytosis or toxic secretions.

Acquired immunity refers to a specific set of events used by the body to fight a particular infection. Essentially, the body accumulates and stores information about the nature of an invading microorganism. As a result, the body can mount a specific attack that is much more effective than innate immunity. It also provides a way for the body to prevent future infections by the same microorganism.

Acquired immunity is divided into a primary response and a secondary response. The **primary immune response** occurs the first time a particular microorganism enters the body, where macrophages engulf the microorganism and travel to the lymph nodes. In the lymph nodes, macrophages present the invader to helper T lymphocytes, which then activate humoral and cellular immunity. Humoral immunity refers to immunity resulting from antibody production by B lymphocytes. After being activated by helper T lymphocytes, B lymphocytes multiply and divide into plasma cells and memory cells. Plasma cells are B lymphocytes that produce immune proteins called antibodies, or immunoglobulins. Antibodies then bind the microorganism to flag it for destruction by other white blood cells. Cellular immunity refers to the immune response coordinated by T lymphocytes. After being activated by helper T lymphocytes, other T lymphocytes attack and kill cells that cause infection or disease.

The **secondary immune response** takes place during subsequent encounters with a known microorganism. Memory cells respond to the previously encountered microorganism by immediately producing antibodies. Memory cells are B lymphocytes that store information to produce antibodies. The secondary immune response is swift and powerful because it eliminates the need for the time-consuming macrophage activation of the primary immune response. Suppressor T lymphocytes also take part to inhibit the immune response, as an overactive immune response could cause damage to healthy cells.

Inflammation occurs if a pathogen evades the barriers and chemical defenses. It stimulates pain receptors, alerting the individual that something is wrong. It also elevates body temperature to speed up chemical reactions, although if a fever goes unchecked it can be dangerous due to the fact that extreme heat unfolds proteins. Histamine is secreted which dilates blood vessels and recruits white blood cells that destroy invaders non-specifically. The immune system is tied to the lymphatic system. The thymus, one of the lymphatic system organs, is the site of maturation of T-cells, a type of white blood cell. The lymphatic system is important in the inflammatory response because lymph vessels deliver leukocytes and collect debris that will be filtered in the lymph nodes and the spleen.

Antigen and Typical Immune Response

Should a pathogen evade barriers and survive through inflammation, an antigen-specific adaptive immune response will begin. Immune cells recognize these foreign particles by their antigens, which are their unique and identifying surface proteins. Drugs, toxins, and transplanted cells can also act as antigens. The body even recognizes its own cells as potential threats in autoimmune diseases.

When a macrophage engulfs a pathogen and presents its antigens, helper T cells recognize the signal and secrete cytokines to signal T lymphocytes and B lymphocytes so that they launch the cell-mediated and humoral response, respectively. The cell-mediated response occurs when the T lymphocytes kill infected cells by secreting cytotoxins. The humoral response occurs when B lymphocytes proliferate into plasma and memory cells. The plasma cells secrete antigen-specific antibodies, which bind to the pathogens so that they cannot bind to host cells. Macrophages and other phagocytic cells called neutrophils engulf and degrade the antibody/pathogen complex. The memory cells remain in circulation and initiate a secondary immune response should the pathogen dare enter the host again.

Active and Passive Immunity

Acquired immunity occurs after the first antigen encounter. The first time the body mounts this immune response is called the primary immune response. Because the memory B cells store information about the antigen's structure, any subsequent immune response causes a secondary immune response, which is much faster and produces substantially more antibodies due to the presence of memory B cells. If the secondary immune response is strong and fast enough, it will fight off the pathogen before an individual becomes symptomatic. This is a natural means of acquiring immunity.

Vaccination is the process of inducing immunity. **Active immunization** refers to immunity gained by exposure to infectious microorganisms or viruses and can be natural or artificial. **Natural immunization** refers to an individual being exposed to an infectious organism as a part of daily life. For example, it was once common for parents to expose their children to childhood diseases such as measles or chicken pox. Artificial immunization refers to therapeutic exposure to an infectious organism as a way of protecting an individual from disease. Today, the medical community relies on artificial immunization as a way to induce immunity.

Vaccines are used for the development of active immunity. A vaccine contains a killed, weakened, or inactivated microorganism or virus that is administered through injection, by mouth, or by aerosol. Vaccinations are administered to prevent an infectious disease but do not always guarantee immunity. Due to circulating memory B cells after administration, the secondary response will fight off the pathogen should it be encountered again in many cases. Both illnesses and vaccinations cause active immunity.

Passive immunity refers to immunity gained by the introduction of antibodies. This introduction can also be natural or artificial. The process occurs when antibodies from the mother's bloodstream are passed on to the bloodstream of the developing fetus. Breast milk can also transmit antibodies to a baby. Babies are born with passive immunity, which provides protection against general infection for approximately the first six months of its life.

Types of Leukocytes

There are many **leukocytes**, or white blood cells, involved in both innate and adaptive immunity. All are developed in bone marrow. Many have been mentioned in the text above, but a comprehensive list is included here for reference.

- Monocytes are large phagocytic cells.
    - Macrophages engulf pathogens and present their antigen. Some circulate, but others reside in lymphatic organs like the spleen and lymph nodes.
    - Dendritic cells are also phagocytic and antigen-presenting.
- Granulocytes are cells that contain secretory granules.
    - Neutrophils are the most abundant white blood cell. They are circulating and aggressive phagocytic cells that are part of innate immunity. They also secrete substances that are toxic to pathogens.
    - Basophils and mast cells secrete histamine, which stimulates the inflammatory response.
    - Eosinophils are found underneath mucous membranes and defend against multicellular parasites like worms. They have low phagocytic activity and primarily secrete destructive enzymes.
- T lymphocytes mature in the thymus.
    - Helper T cells recognize antigens presented by macrophages and dendritic cells and secrete cytokines, which mount the humoral and cell-mediated immune response.
    - Killer T cells are cytotoxic cells involved in the cell-mediated response by recognizing and poisoning infected cells.
    - Suppressor T cells suppress the adaptive immune response when there is no threat to conserve resources and energy.
    - Memory T cells remain in circulation to aid in the secondary immune response.
- B lymphocytes mature in bone marrow.
    - Plasma B cells secrete antigen-specific antibodies when signaled by Helper T cells and are degraded after the immune response.
    - Memory B cells store antigen-specific antibody making instructions and remain circulating after the immune response is over.
- Natural killer cells are part of innate immunity and patrol and identify suspect-material. They respond by secreting cytotoxic substances.

Neurology

The human **nervous system** coordinates the body's response to stimuli from inside and outside the body. There are two major types of nervous system cells: neurons and neuroglia. **Neurons** are the workhorses of the nervous system and form a complex communication network that transmits electrical impulses termed **action potentials**, while **neuroglia** connect and support the neurons. Motor neurons use sodium and potassium pumps and channels in order to make action potentials occur.

Although some neurons monitor the senses, some control muscles, and some connect the brain to other neurons, all neurons have four common characteristics:

- **Dendrites**: These receive electrical signals from other neurons across small gaps called *synapses*.
- **Nerve cell body**: This is the hub of processing and protein manufacture for the neuron.
- **Axon**: This transmits the signal from the cell body to other neurons.
- **Terminals**: These bridge the neuron to dendrites of other neurons and deliver the signal via chemical messengers called **neurotransmitters**.

Here is an illustration of this:

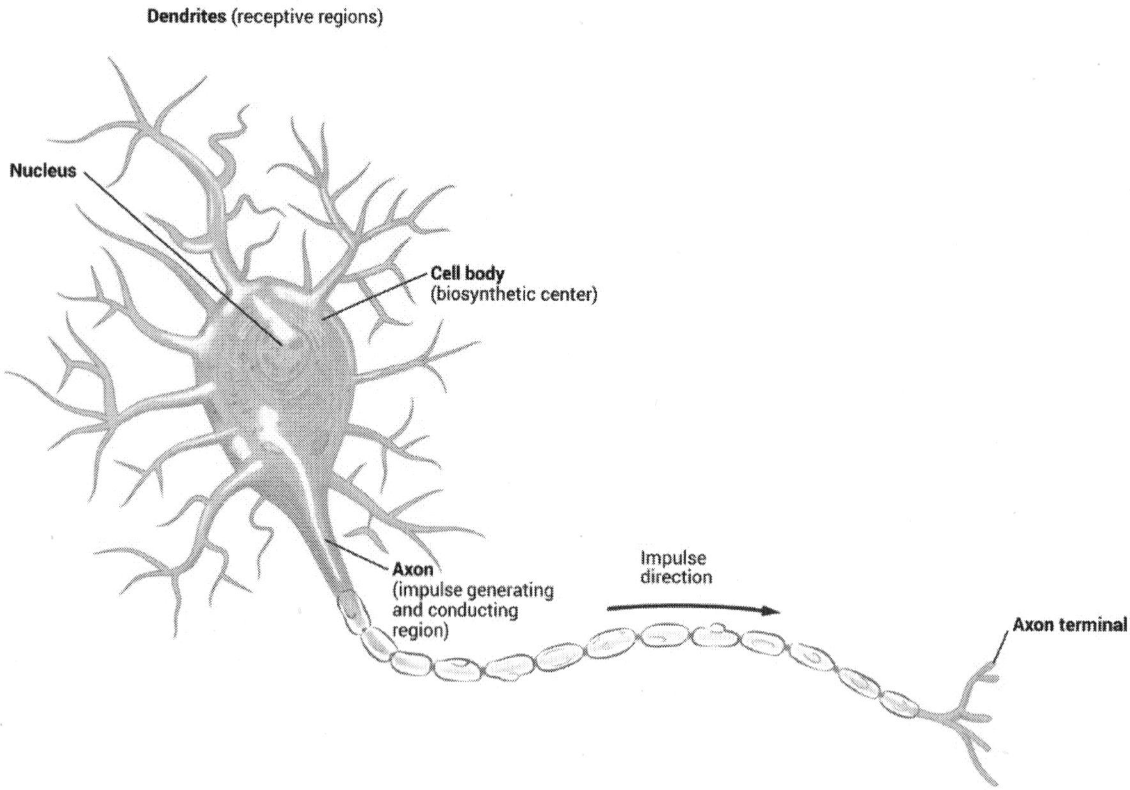

There are two major divisions of the nervous system: central and peripheral.

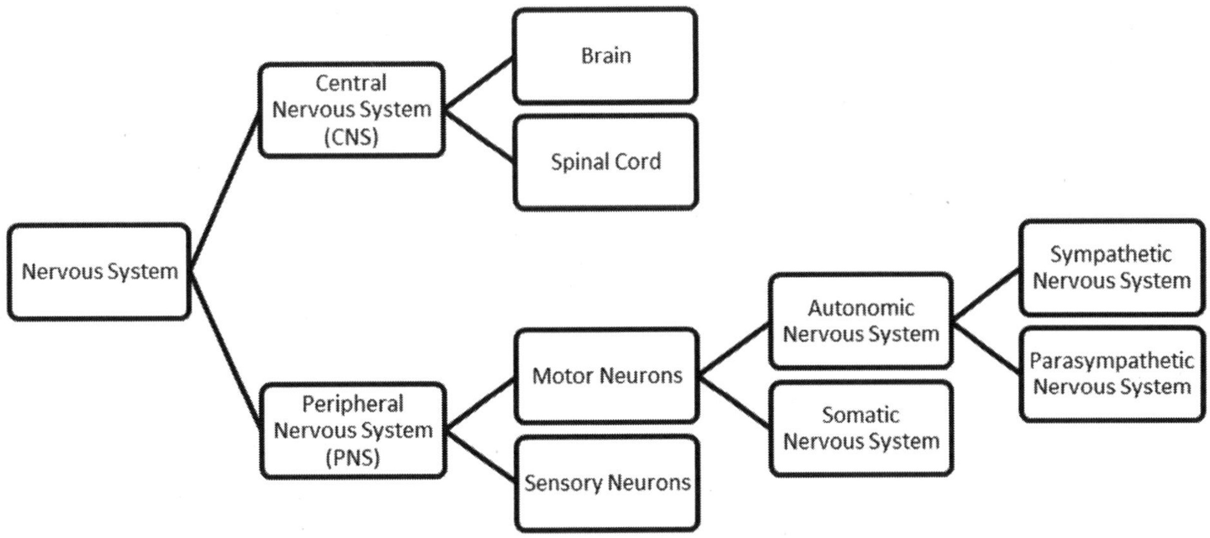

Central Nervous System

The **central nervous system (CNS)** consists of the brain and spinal cord. Three layers of membranes called the meninges cover and separate the CNS from the rest of the body.

The major divisions of the brain are the forebrain, the midbrain, and the hindbrain.

The **forebrain** consists of the cerebrum, the thalamus and hypothalamus, and the rest of the limbic system. The **cerebrum** is the largest part of the brain, and its most well-documented part is the outer cerebral cortex. The cerebrum is divided into right and left hemispheres, and each cerebral cortex hemisphere has four discrete areas, or lobes: frontal, temporal, parietal, and occipital.

The **frontal lobe** governs duties such as voluntary movement, judgment, problem solving, and planning, while the other lobes are more sensory. The **temporal lobe** integrates hearing and language comprehension, the **parietal lobe** processes sensory input from the skin, and the **occipital** lobe processes visual input from the eyes. For completeness, the other two senses, smell and taste, are processed via the olfactory bulbs. The thalamus helps organize and coordinate all of this sensory input in a meaningful way for the brain to interpret.

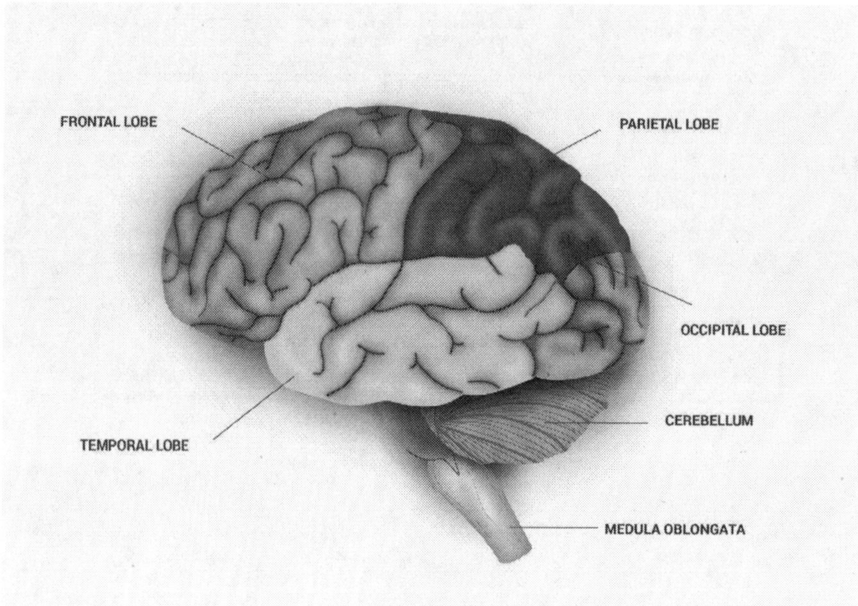

The **hypothalamus** controls the endocrine system and all of the hormones that govern long-term effects on the body. Each hemisphere of the limbic system includes a **hippocampus** (which plays a vital role in memory), an **amygdala** (which is involved with emotional responses like fear and anger), and other small bodies and nuclei associated with memory and pleasure.

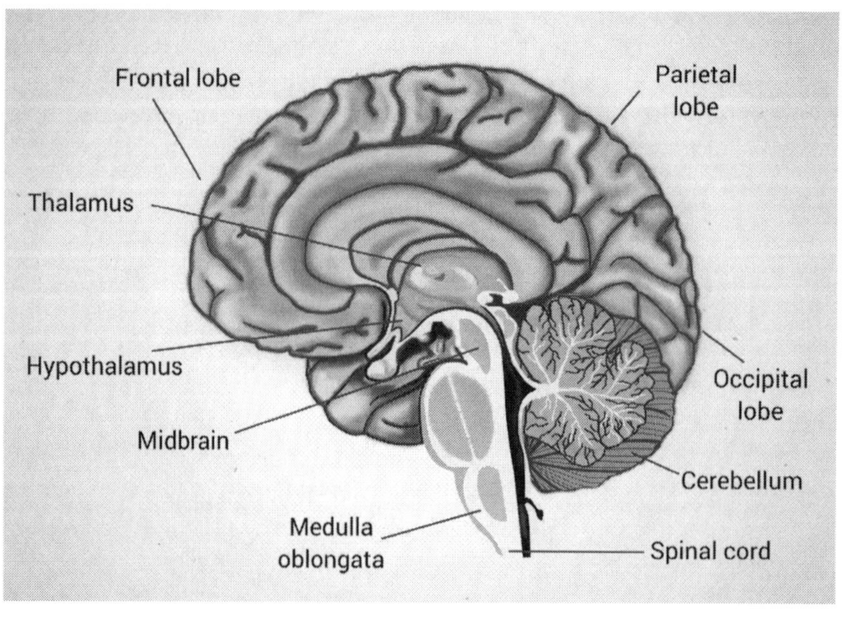

The **midbrain** is in charge of alertness, sleep/wake cycles, and temperature regulation, and it includes the **substantia nigra** which produces melatonin to regulate sleep patterns. The notable components of the **hindbrain** include the **medulla oblongata** and **cerebellum**. The **medulla oblongata** is located just above the spinal cord and is responsible for crucial involuntary functions such as breathing, swallowing, and regulating heart rate and blood pressure. Together with other parts of the hindbrain, the midbrain and medulla oblongata form the **brain stem**. The brain stem connects the spinal cord to the rest of the brain. To the rear of the brain stem sits the cerebellum, which plays key roles in posture, balance, and muscular coordination. The spinal cord itself, which is encapsulated by the protective bony spinal column, carries sensory information to the brain and motor information to the body.

Peripheral Nervous System

The **peripheral nervous system (PNS)** includes all nervous tissue besides the brain and spinal cord. The PNS consists of the sets of cranial and spinal nerves and relays information between the CNS and the rest of the body. The PNS has two divisions: the autonomic nervous system and the somatic nervous system.

Autonomic Nervous System

The **autonomic nervous system (ANS)** governs involuntary, or reflexive, body functions. Ultimately, the autonomic nervous system controls functions such as breathing, heart rate, digestion, body temperature, and blood pressure.

The ANS is split between parasympathetic nerves and sympathetic nerves. These two nerve types are antagonistic and have opposite effects on the body. Parasympathetic nerves predominate resting conditions, and decrease heart rate, decrease breathing rate, prepare digestion, and allow urination and excretion. **Sympathetic nerves**, on the other hand, become active when a person is under stress or excited, and they increase heart rate, increase breathing rates, and inhibit digestion, urination, and excretion.

Somatic Nervous System and the Reflex Arc

The **somatic nervous system (SNS)** governs the conscious, or voluntary, control of skeletal muscles and their corresponding body movements. The SNS contains afferent and efferent neurons. **Afferent neurons** carry sensory messages from the skeletal muscles, skin, or sensory organs to the CNS. **Efferent neurons** relay motor messages from the CNS to skeletal muscles, skin, or sensory organs.

The SNS also has a role in involuntary movements called **reflexes**. A reflex is defined as an involuntary response to a stimulus. They are transmitted via what is termed a **reflex arc**, where a stimulus is sensed by an affector and its afferent neuron, interpreted and rerouted by an interneuron, and delivered to effector muscles by an efferent neuron where they respond to the initial stimulus. A reflex is able to bypass the brain by being rerouted through the spinal cord; the interneuron decides the proper course of action rather than the brain. The reflex arc results in an instantaneous, involuntary response. For example, a physician tapping on the knee produces an involuntary knee jerk referred to as the patellar tendon reflex.

Renal System

The **renal system** or **urinary system** is made up of the kidneys, ureters, urinary bladder, and the urethra. It is the system responsible for removing waste products and balancing water and electrolyte concentrations in the blood. The urinary system has many important functions related to waste excretion. It regulates the concentrations of sodium, potassium, chloride, calcium, and other ions in the filtrate by controlling the amount of each that is reabsorbed during filtration. The reabsorption or secretion of hydrogen ions and bicarbonate contributes to the maintenance of blood pH. Certain kidney cells can detect any reductions in blood volume and pressure. If that happens, they secrete renin, which activates a hormone that causes increased reabsorption of sodium ions and water, raising volume and pressure. Under hypoxic conditions, kidney cells will secrete erythropoietin in order to stimulate red blood cell production. Kidney cells also synthesize **calcitriol**, which is a hormone derivative of vitamin D3 that aids in calcium ion absorption by the intestinal epithelium.

Under normal circumstances, humans have two functioning **kidneys** in the lower back and on either side of the spinal cord. They are the main organs that are responsible for filtering waste products out of the blood and regulating blood water and electrolyte levels. Blood enters the kidney through the renal artery, and urea and wastes are removed, while water and the acidity/alkalinity of the blood is adjusted. Toxic substances and drugs are also filtered. Blood exits through the renal vein, and the urine waste travels through the ureter to the bladder, where it is stored until it is eliminated through the urethra.

The kidneys have an outer renal cortex and an inner renal medulla that contain millions of tiny filtering units called **nephrons**. Nephrons have two parts: a glomerulus, which is the filter, and a tubule. The **glomerulus** is a network of capillaries covered by the **Bowman's capsule**, which is the entrance to the tubule. As blood enters the kidneys via the renal artery, the glomerulus allows for fluid and waste products to pass through it and enter the tubule. Blood cells and large molecules, such as proteins, do not pass through and remain in the blood. The **filtrate** passes through the tubule, which has several parts.

The proximal tubule comes first, and then the descending and ascending limbs of the loop of Henle dip into the medulla, followed by the distal tubule and collecting duct. The journey through the tubule involves a balancing act that regulates blood osmolarity, pH, and electrolytes exchange of materials between the tubule and the bloodstream. The final product at the collecting tubule is called urine, and it is delivered to the bladder by the ureter. The most central part of the kidney is the **renal pelvis**, and it acts as a funnel by delivering the urine from the millions of collecting tubules to the **ureters**. The filtered blood exits through the renal vein and is returned to circulation.

Here's a look at the genitourinary system:

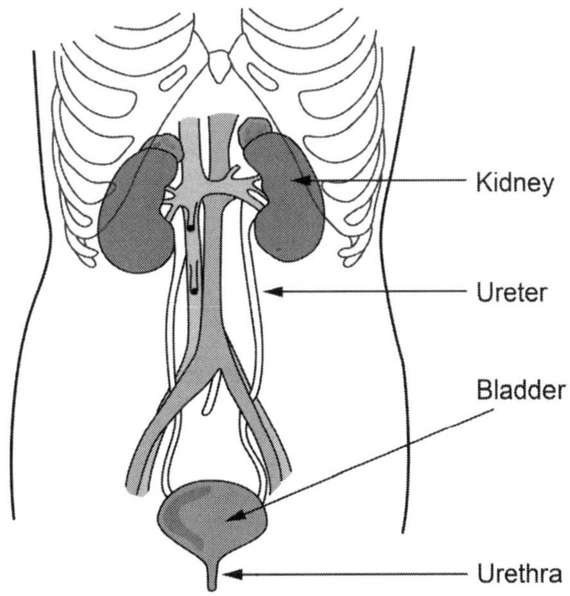

Here's a close up look at the kidney:

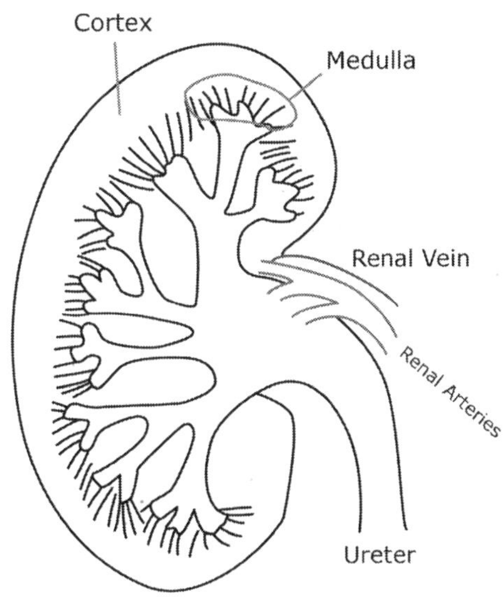

Waste Excretion

Once urine accumulates, it leaves the kidneys. The urine travels through the ureters into the **urinary bladder**, a muscular organ that is hollow and elastic. As more urine enters the urinary bladder, its walls stretch and become thinner so there is no significant difference in internal pressure. The urinary bladder stores the urine until the body is ready for urination, at which time the muscles contract and force the urine through the **urethra** and out of the body.

Hematological System

The hematological system consists of the components of blood and the structures that form them, such as bone marrow and the spleen.

Blood is vital to the human body. It is a liquid connective tissue that serves as a transport system for supplying cells with nutrients and carrying away their wastes. The average adult human has five to six quarts of blood circulating through their body. Approximately 55% of blood is plasma (the fluid portion), and the remaining 45% is composed of solid cells and cell parts. There are three major types of blood cells:

- **Red blood cells**, or **erythrocytes**, transport oxygen throughout the body. They contain a protein called **hemoglobin** that allows them to carry oxygen. The iron in the hemoglobin gives the cells and the blood their red colors.
- **White blood cells**, or **leukocytes**, are responsible for fighting infectious diseases and maintaining the immune system. Monocytes, lymphocytes (including B-cells and T-cells), neutrophils, basophils, and eosinophils compose the white blood cells. All are developed in bone marrow. **Monocytes** eat and destroy invaders like bacteria and viruses. **Lymphocytes** are responsible for antibody creation in the defense against invasive organisms and infections. **Neutrophils**, the most abundant white blood cell, take out bacterial and fungal organisms. They are the first line of defense against infections. **Basophils** and mast cells secrete histamine, the substance responsible for itching associated with allergic diseases. **Eosinophils** target parasites and cancer cells and are part of the body's allergic response. They have low phagocytic activity and primarily secrete destructive enzymes.
- Platelets are cell fragments that play a central role in the blood clotting process.

All blood cells in adults are produced in the bone marrow—red blood cells and most white blood cells are produced in the red marrow, and some white blood cells are produced in the yellow bone marrow.

Blood type is a trait that has multiple alleles: I^A, I^B, and i. I^A and I^B are co-dominant so neither is "stronger" than the other, and i is recessive to both. In the event that both co-dominant alleles are present in a genotype, both phenotypes will be present.

Genotype	Phenotype	Blood Donation Facts
IAIA, IAi	A blood (A antigens and B antibodies)	People with A blood can't receive blood from AB or B due to antibody recognition and attack of B antigen.
IAIB	AB blood (A and B antigens but no antibodies)	Universal receiver because it contains no antibodies against A or B antigens.
IBIB, IBi	B blood (B antigens and A antibodies)	People with B blood can't receive blood from AB or A due to antibody recognition and attack of A antigen.
Ii	O blood (A and B antibodies)	Can only receive from other O blood (universal donor).

Blood type demonstrates the concept of co-dominance as well as multiple alleles. Below are some blood type crosses and probabilities.

$I^A I^A$ x $I^A i$

	I^A	I^A
I^A	$I^A I^A$ A blood	$I^A I^A$ A blood
i	$I^A i$ A blood	$I^A i$ A blood

$I^A i$ x $I^A i$

	I^A	i
I^A	$I^A I^A$ A blood	$I^A i$ A blood
i	$I^A i$ A blood	$i i$ 0 blood

Closely tied to the hematological system is the **lymphatic system**. Like the circulatory and hematological systems, the lymphatic system is a network of vessels and organs that move fluid—in this case, lymph—throughout the body. The lymphatic system works in concert with the immune system to help the body process toxins and waste. **Lymph** has a high concentration of white blood cells, which help attack viruses and bacteria throughout body cells and tissues. Lymph is filtered in nodes along the vessels; the body has 600 to 700 lymph nodes, which may be superficial (like those in the armpit and groin) or deep (such as those around the heart and lungs). The spleen is the largest organ of the lymphatic system and it helps produce the lymphocytes (white blood cells) to control infections. It also controls the number of red blood cells in the body. Other lymphatic organs include the tonsils, adenoids, and thymus.

Homeostasis

In order for organisms to survive against this universal tendency for chaos, they must use energy to work against entropy. They do this via biochemical processes that maintain an internal order, called homeostasis. **Homeostasis** is the physiological processes within a system that regulate a stable internal equilibrium such as body temperature, blood pH, and fluid balance.

An example of homeostasis in the human body is temperature regulation. The skin has a thermoregulatory role in the human body that is controlled by a negative feedback loop. The control center of temperature regulation is the hypothalamus in the brain. When the hypothalamus is alerted by receptors from the dermis, it secretes hormones that activate effectors to keep internal temperature at a set point of 98.6°F (37°C). If the environment is too cold, the hypothalamus will initiate a pathway that induces muscle shivering to release heat energy as well as constrict blood vessels to limit heat loss. In hot conditions, the hypothalamus will initiate a pathway that vasodilates blood vessels to increase heat loss and stimulate sweating for evaporative cooling. Evaporative cooling occurs when the hottest water particles evaporate and leave behind the coolest ones. This cools down the body.

Organisms maintain homeostasis by using free energy and matter, usually in the form of atoms and molecules. Atoms are the smallest whole units of matter, and molecules are atoms connected to each other via chemical bonds. Everything is made up of atoms, even the most complicated structures; their complexity is only due to the variety and quantity of different molecular arrangements. A famous experiment by Stanley Miller and Harold Urey simulated early Earth's atmospheric conditions and witnessed the synthesis of a string of molecules known as amino acids. **Amino acids** are the blueprints of proteins—the building blocks of life. This famous experiment provided a glimpse of the original atomic arrangements that facilitated the origin of life. Before proteins, random particles would collide, due to chance, only if given enough time. After proteins arrived, life arose, likely because proteins enable organisms to use available energy and matter to make complicated structures, from cells to whole organisms. **Enzymes** (proteins that act as catalysts) help reactants find each other by providing a docking station, increasing probabilities of atomic collision and bonding, and therefore, facilitate the specific biochemical reactions that make life possible.

Here's an illustration of that:

The Lock and Key Mechanism

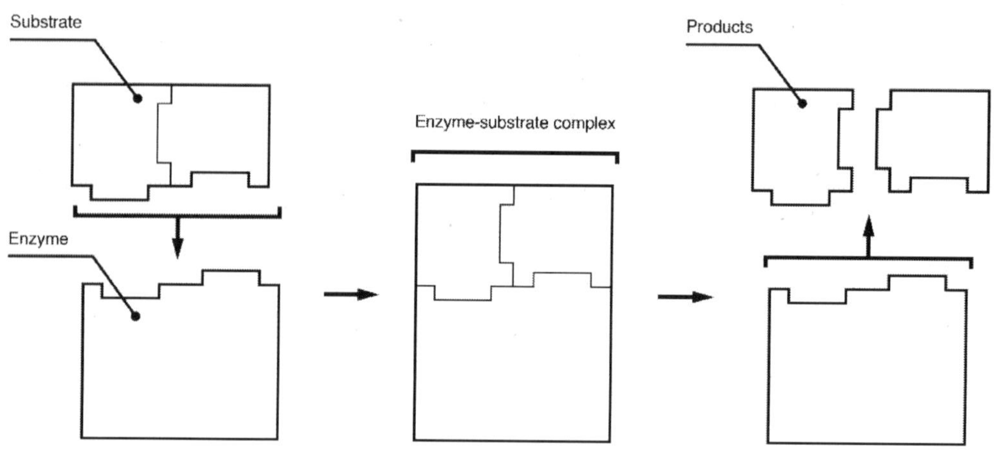

Proteins combine to make a myriad of different structures. Think of proteins like people. A pile of bricks can't do anything on its own. Buildings can only form when there are workers to move the bricks into place. Similarly, proteins turn matter into the complicated structures that form organisms.

Proteins in the form of enzymes are especially important for biochemical reactions because they lower the activation energy—the minimum energy required for a chemical reaction to happen—as illustrated in the below graph.

Using available free energy, reactions occur within an organism that create organization and decrease entropy. The below graphs illustrate how free energy is used in two basic biochemical reactions:

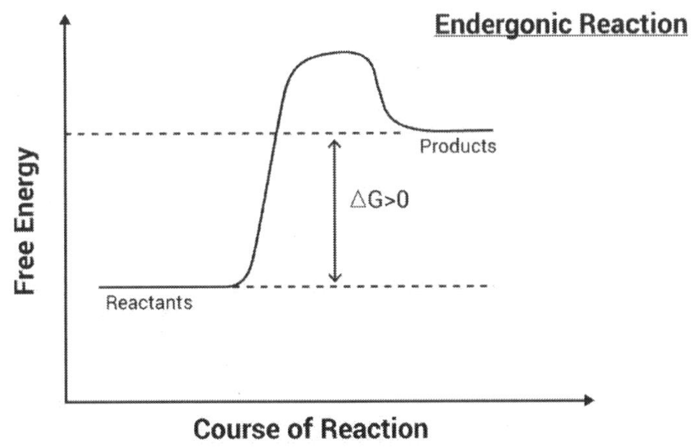

The image above illustrates a reaction that decreases entropy (or increases order), called an **endergonic reaction**. Endergonic, or anabolic, reactions occur when reactants absorb energy from the surroundings so that the products hold more energy than the reactants. Anabolic reactions enable the organism to make bigger things (polymers) from smaller things (monomers), such as forming new cells, or making proteins from amino acids.

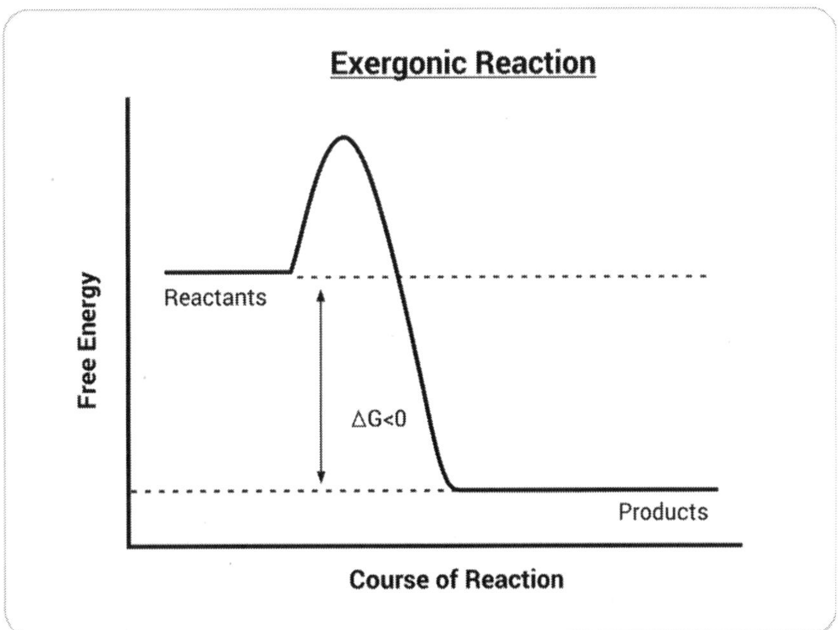

Conversely, the image above illustrates an exergonic, or catabolic, reaction that releases energy. In this reaction, the products hold less energy than the reactants, and entropy (or disorder) is increased. Catabolic reactions enable organisms to break down bigger things (polymers) into smaller things (monomers); for example, breaking down proteins into their respective amino acids.

As long as the energy released (exergonic) exceeds the energy absorbed (endergonic) in an organism, it will continue to function and sustain life. If there is not energy available from exergonic reactions to drive endergonic reactions, the organism will die, since energy is required to perform all metabolic functions. Metabolism is the set of processes carried out by an organism that permits the exchange of energy between itself and the environment, enabling it to change and grow internally.

In other words: metabolism = catabolism + anabolism

- If catabolism is greater than anabolism, i.e., energy released is greater than energy consumed, then an organism can live.
- If catabolism is less than anabolism, i.e., energy released is less than energy consumed, then an organism will die.

Organisms must consume energy, in the form of food or light, to perform anabolic reactions. If they are autotrophs, such as plants, they produce their own food. If they are heterotrophs, such as animals, they absorb the energy provided by food, most commonly sugars. The most common form of sugar used for energy is the simple sugar glucose, $C_6H_{12}O_6$, which contains extremely high amounts of potential energy stored within its atomic bonds.

Feedback Mechanisms

Like most organisms, humans regulate cellular processes through feedback loops to fine-tune many other processes, including water osmolarity.

In blood, **osmolarity** refers to the concentration of the collective solutes and water in the blood, and it is regulated by the hypothalamus. The **hypothalamus** is the bridge between the nervous and endocrine systems via the pituitary gland, and it contains osmoreceptors that sense blood osmolarity. If blood has a low percentage of water, then an individual is dehydrated and has high blood osmolarity. If osmolarity is high, the hypothalamus stimulates the pituitary gland to release stored antidiuretic hormone (ADH). ADH stimulates the kidneys to increase water permeability in the collecting ducts, which increases reabsorption of water and reduces urine volume, meaning less water is lost through urination. This water-retaining mechanism will eventually lower the osmolarity, and when it falls below its set point, osmoreceptors will inhibit the hypothalamus from initiating reabsorption.

This is an example of a negative feedback loop because the stimulus feeds back to the regulator in order to change the production in the opposite direction. If production is too high, the system turns off, and if production is too low, the system turns on. Negative feedback loops respond to environmental conditions to keep them at a "set point."

Positive feedback loops also exist to amplify responses in the presence of production, such as with intracellular signaling cascades or recruitment of cells in the immune system. They do not necessarily ensure cellular homeostasis, but rather they ensure functionality. For example, the production of oxytocin during childbirth is a critical positive feedback loop. In the case of childbirth, the initial stimulus is pressure on the cervix, which sends a message to the brain that causes the pituitary gland to secrete oxytocin, which acts on the uterus to stimulate contractions. As the pressure on the cervix increases, more oxytocin is produced in a positive feedback cycle. Once the baby and placenta are delivered, pressure on the cervix disappears, the pituitary stops producing oxytocin, and uterine contractions stop. Without this positive feedback loop, it would be impossible to provide the force necessary to deliver babies vaginally.

Non-functional feedback loops can be deadly. The classic example is type I diabetes, in which there is an autoimmune response against the beta cells of the pancreas, the insulin-producing cells.

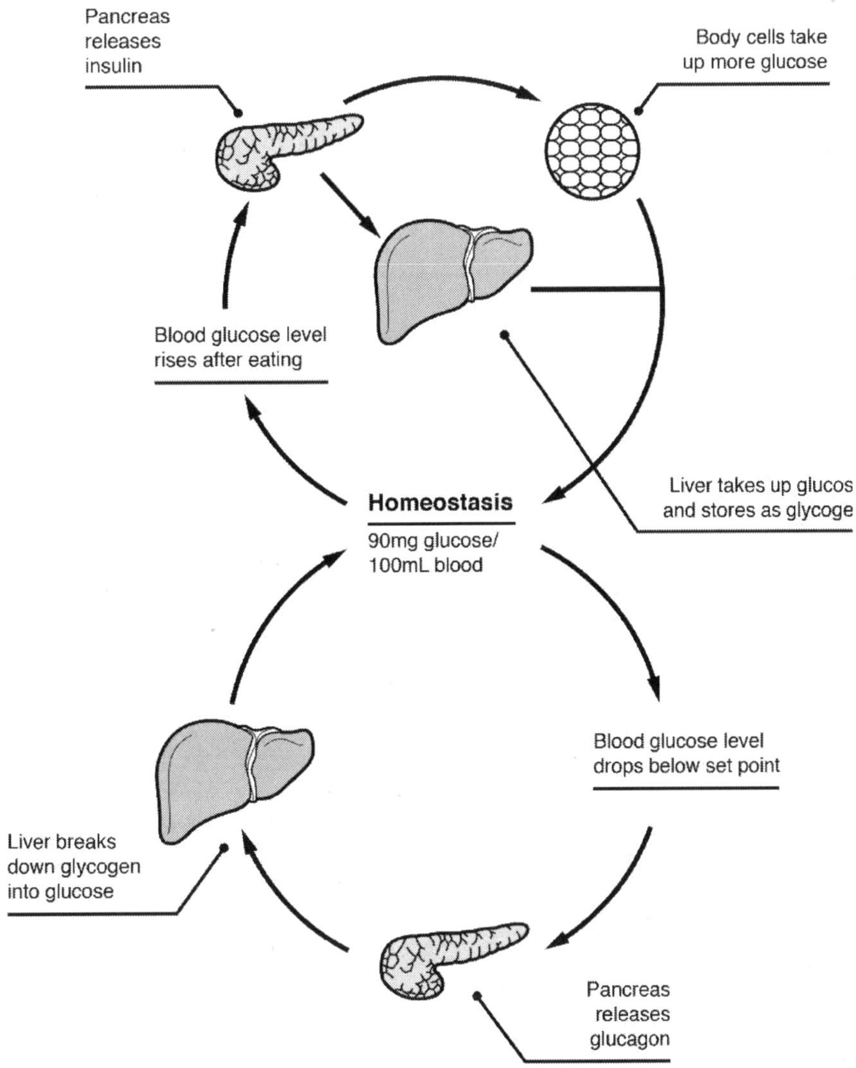

The balance between insulin and glucagon is disrupted when the pancreas can't produce insulin. Insulin serves to open the carrier proteins on cellular membranes, allowing glucose entry. In the absence of insulin, the carrier proteins in cells are not signaled to take in glucose, causing blood sugar to rise. In normal, healthy conditions, in response to high blood sugar, the pancreas is stimulated to produce more insulin from the beta cells (specialized insulin-producing cells). In diabetics, the beta cells have been destroyed by the autoimmune system. The whole bottom portion of the feedback loop is bypassed, and as a result, diabetics become severely hyperglycemic without artificial insulin administration. Severe hyperglycemia can result in coma and death.

Respiratory System

The **respiratory system** enables breathing and supports the energy-making process in cells. The respiratory system transports an essential reactant, oxygen, to cells so that they can produce energy in their mitochondria via cellular respiration. The respiratory system also removes carbon dioxide, a waste product of cellular respiration.

This system is divided into the upper respiratory system and the lower respiratory system. The **upper respiratory system** comprises the nose, the nasal cavity and sinuses, and the pharynx. The **lower respiratory system** comprises the larynx (voice box), the trachea (windpipe), the small passageways leading to the lungs, and the lungs.

The pathway of oxygen to the bloodstream begins with the nose and the mouth. Upon inhalation, air enters the nose and mouth and passes into the sinuses where it gets warmed, filtered, and humidified. The throat, or the pharynx, allows the entry of both food and air; however, only air moves into the trachea, or windpipe, since the epiglottis covers the trachea during swallowing and prevents food from entering. The trachea contains mucus and cilia. The mucus traps many airborne pathogens while the cilia act as bristles that sweep the pathogens away toward the top of the trachea where they are either swallowed or coughed out.

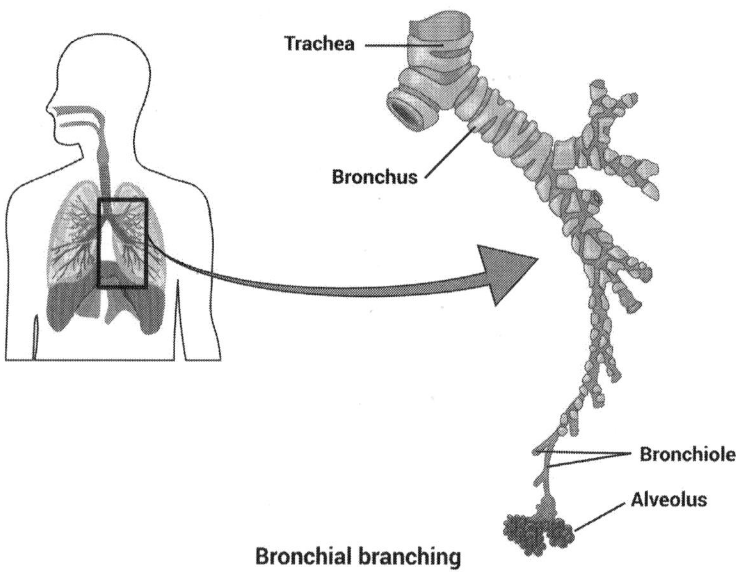

Bronchial branching

The **trachea** itself has two vocal cords at the top that make up the larynx. At its bottom, the trachea forks into two major bronchi—one for each lung. These bronchi continue to branch into smaller and smaller bronchioles before terminating in grape-like air sacs called **alveoli**; these alveoli are surrounded by capillaries and provide the body with an enormous amount of surface area to exchange oxygen and carbon dioxide gases, in a process called **external respiration**.

In total, the lungs contain about 1,500 miles of airway passages. The right lung is divided into three lobes (superior, middle, and inferior), and the left lung is divided into two lobes (superior and inferior).

The left lung is smaller than the right lung, likely because it shares its space in the chest cavity with the heart.

A flat muscle underneath the lungs called the **diaphragm** controls breathing. When the diaphragm contracts, the volume of the chest cavity increases and indirectly decreases its air pressure. This decrease in air pressure creates a vacuum, and the lungs pull in air to fill the space. This difference in air pressure pulls the air from outside of the body into the lungs in a process called negative pressure breathing.

Upon inhalation or inspiration, oxygen in the alveoli diffuses into the capillaries to be carried by blood to cells throughout the body, in a process called **internal respiration**. A protein called hemoglobin in red blood cells easily bonds with oxygen, removing it from the blood and allowing more oxygen to diffuse in. This protein allows the blood to take in 60 times more oxygen than the body could without it, and this explains how oxygen can become so concentrated in blood even though it is only 21% of the atmosphere. While oxygen diffuses from the alveoli into the capillaries, carbon dioxide diffuses from the capillaries into the alveoli. When the diaphragm relaxes, the elastic lungs snap back to their original shape; this decreases the volume of the chest cavity and increases the air pressure until it is back to normal. This increased air pressure pushes the carbon dioxide waste from the alveoli through exhalation or expiration.

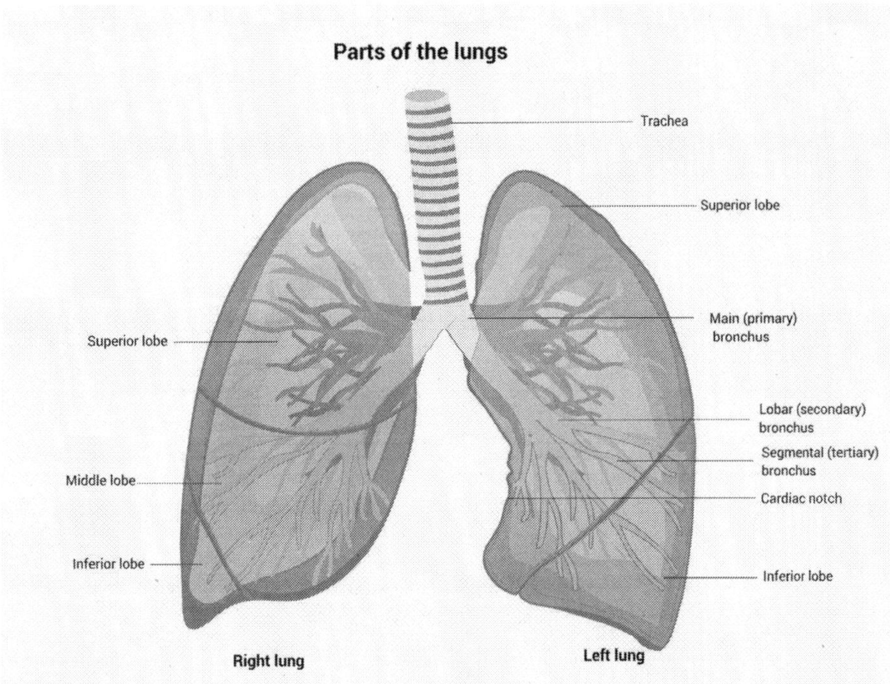

The autonomic nervous system controls breathing. The medulla oblongata gets feedback regarding the carbon dioxide levels in the blood and will send a message to the diaphragm that it is time for a contraction. While breathing can be voluntary, it is mostly under autonomic control.

Functions of the Respiratory System

The respiratory system has many functions. Most importantly, it provides a large area for gas exchange between the air and the circulating blood. It protects the delicate respiratory surfaces from environmental variations and defends them against pathogens. It is responsible for producing the sounds that the body makes for speaking and singing, as well as for non-verbal communication. It also helps regulate blood volume and blood pressure by releasing vasopressin, and it is a regulator of blood pH due to its control over carbon dioxide release, as the aqueous form of carbon dioxide is the chief buffering agent in blood. Erythrocytes use carbonic anhydrase to convert most carbon dioxide in the blood to bicarbonate ions.

Sensory System

Humans understand the world around them through sensory processing. The human body has receptors that sense or detect different types of energy or stimuli and then process that information through the nervous system. This is the simplified process of sensation, such as that involved in touch and smell. The energy is converted to electrical signals and then transmitted to the brain through a series of action potentials travelling along the axons of millions of neural cells.

The **sensory threshold** is the amount or level of stimulus that is required for an individual to register a sensation. The absolute threshold refers to the smallest detectable level of any kind of sensory stimulus that an individual can detect 50% of the time during a given test. The **difference threshold** is the smallest difference between two stimuli that an individual can actually detect as being different 50% of the time during a given test.

The process of **signal detection** occurs when someone detects a stimulus and must distinguish it from background noise. Signal detection theory states that how an individual perceives a stimulus depends on the individual's physical and psychological state, as well as the intensity of the stimulus. For example, in a crowded parking lot, an individual may not notice the rustling of leaves on the ground, but on a quiet day, the sound of the rustling leaves would be more apparent and the individual may pay more attention to it, since there are fewer background noises.

Sensory Receptors

Different types of sensory receptors recognize different types of energy. For example, light receptors, which are located in the eyes, and sound receptors, which are located in the ears, convert their respective energy stimuli to neural activity through different specialized pathways.

Different types of sensations are processed by different sensory receptors. Below is a list of the main sensory receptors found in the human body.

- **Mechanoreceptors**: Detect touch through contact with the body surface and detect sound through vibrations in the air or water. They are located in the skin, hair follicles, and ligaments.
- **Photoreceptors**: Detect vision through visible radiant energy
- **Thermoreceptors**: Detect warmth and cold through changes in skin temperature
- **Chemoreceptors**: Detect smell through substances dissolved in the air or water through the nasal cavity, and taste through substances that come in contact with the tongue

Sensory Pathways

Each type of stimuli, such as touch, hearing, and vision, follows a different sensory pathway from the receptor to the brain. However, generally, all pathways have three long neurons called the primary, secondary, and tertiary neurons. The **primary neuron** has its cell body in the dorsal root ganglion of the spinal nerve. The **secondary neuron** has its cell body either in the spinal cord or in the brain stem. The **tertiary neuron** has its cell body in the thalamus. The pathway includes many breakpoints, or stations, each of which plays a different role in information processing. For example, if a painful sensation is felt on the finger, one station may cause the hand to withdraw from the stimuli and another station may cause the head to turn towards the source of the pain.

Vision

The **eye** is an elaborate organ that allows individuals to transduce light into neural signals and process their surrounding environment. Depending on their level of focus and concentration on an image, humans can see more or less detail on that object. The eye has many features that are similar to those of a camera. The **lens** allows the eye to focus light. The **ciliary muscles** bend the lens to change its shape and adjust the focus. The **cornea** is curved and bends the light rays so that they can form an image on the **retina** in the back of the eye. The amount of light that enters the eye is controlled by the **pupil**. The **optic nerve**, which is made up of the axons from the ganglion cells in the eye, then conveys the visual information to the brain.

Diagram of the Eye

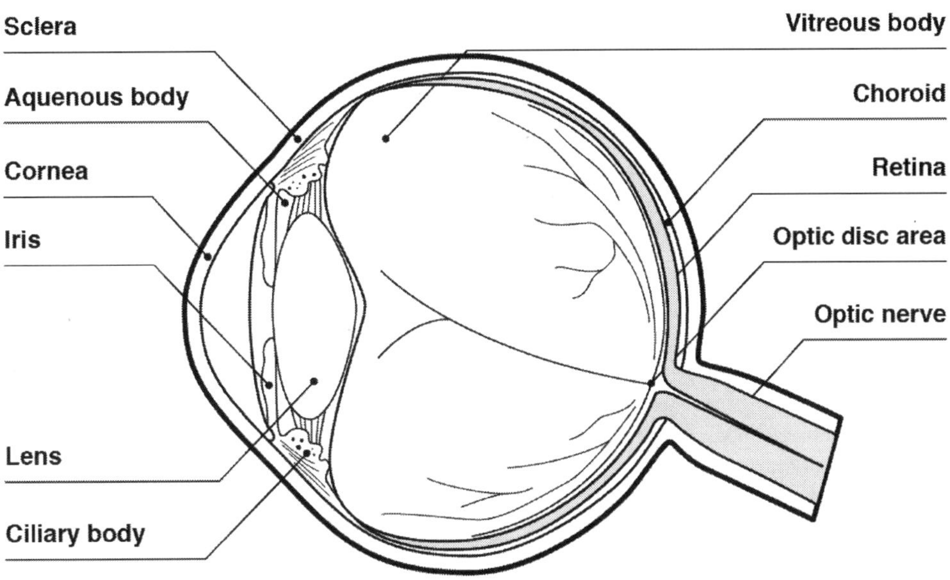

Visual processing begins in the retina. Images that are taken in through the cornea and lens are transmitted upside down onto the retina. The two types of photoreceptors in the retina are called rods and cones. **Rods** are part of the scotopic system and can be stimulated with low light intensity. **Cones** are part of the photopic system and need strong light intensity to be stimulated. The **photopic system** is responsible for color vision. The signals that are produced from the processing that occurs in the retina are then transferred to ganglion cells, whose axons make up the optic nerve. Signals travel along these axons to the brain, where the visual information is processed, and the images are returned to their proper orientation.

Visual Pathways in the Brain

An individual's visual field is the entire area that they can see without moving their head. The visual cortex in the right hemisphere of the brain receives its input from the left half of the visual field and the visual cortex in the left hemisphere of the brain receives its input from the right half of the visual field. Some retinal ganglion cells have axons that lead to the superior colliculus in the brain, which helps coordinate the rapid movements of the eye towards a target. Others have axons that lead to the nuclei of the hypothalamus that control **circadian rhythms**, or the daily cycles of human behavior, or to the midbrain nuclei to control the size of the pupil and coordinate movement of the eyes or to map the visual space.

Parallel Processing

Parallel processing is the method by which the brain distinguishes incoming stimuli of differing quality. When processing visual stimuli, the brain divides what it sees into the categories of color, motion, shape, and depth. Each quality is analyzed individually, but simultaneously, and then combined together for comprehension of the object.

Feature Detection

Feature detection is a process that starts gradually when an individual begins looking at an object. At first, the individual may look at the overall object, but as the neurons in the brain become more focused on the object, smaller details become more apparent. Feature detection allows the brain to become more selective in what it focuses on. For example, from a picture of a woman's face, the brain begins to see the curves, angles, and small lines of the face as the individual looks at the picture for a longer time.

Hearing

Diagram of the Ear

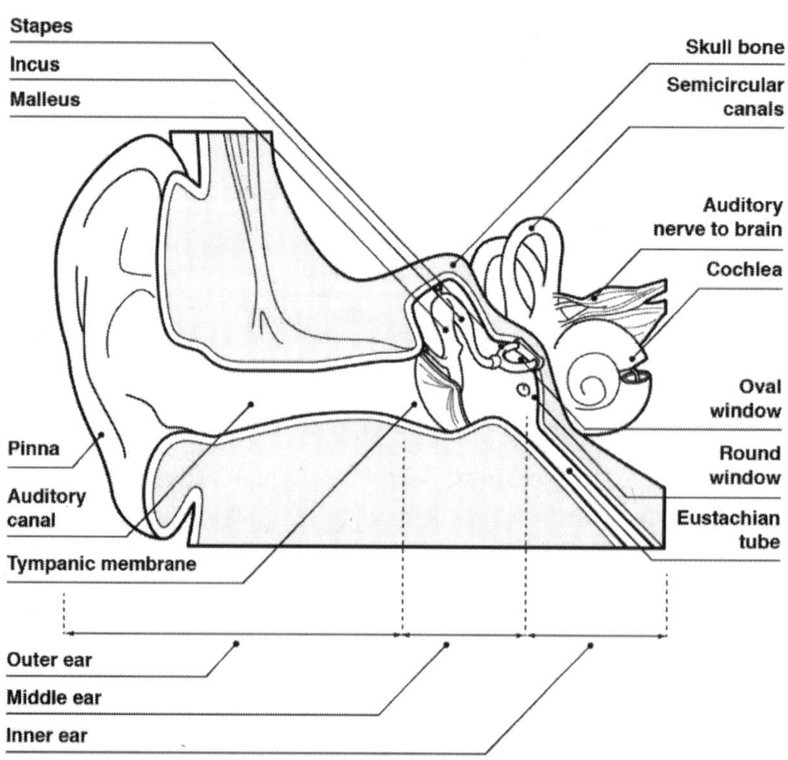

Each part of the ear plays a specific role in hearing. The **external ear** captures sound waves and sends them down the ear canal to the eardrum, or tympanic membrane. The shape of the external ear is important because it increases the efficiency of sounds within a certain frequency, especially those within the range important for speech perception, and helps with sound localization, so that individuals can identify where a sound is coming from. The **middle ear** consists of a chain of three small bones called **ossicles** that connect the tympanic membrane to the **oval window**, which is the opening of the inner ear. The ossicles are responsible for transferring and concentrating the mechanical stimuli of the tympanic membrane through the fluid of the middle ear to the auditory portion of the inner ear, which is called the **cochlea**. The inner ear has a structure called the **organ of Corti** that then converts the sound energy into neural activity. The organ of Corti has hairs on it that either convey messages to the brain or receive messages back from the brain.

Once a sound reaches the organ of Corti, it then travels as an electrical signal through the auditory ganglion cells and afferent nerves to the cochlear nuclei in the brainstem. There is a cochlear nucleus on each side of the brainstem, one for each ear. The signal then reaches the **superior olivary nuclei**, which is the first location to receive signals from both ears. This helps greatly with auditory localization. Signals then travel to the inferior colliculus, the medial geniculate nucleus, and then to the auditory cortex. The neurons on this pathway are arranged in a very organized manner, dependent on the stimuli that they process. For example, cells that respond to high frequency sounds are at a distance from those that respond to low frequency sounds.

Each ear contains about 3,500 inner hair cells (IHCs) and 12,000 outer hair cells (OHCs). IHCs cannot regenerate, so damage to them causes a permanent decrease in hearing sensitivity. The IHC and OHC each have about 50 to 200 **stereocilia**, which are even smaller, stiff hairs protruding from them. Approximately 16 to 20 auditory nerve fibers come in contact with each IHC. The organ of Corti has two **afferent** nerve fibers, whose job is to convey messages from the hair cells to the brain, and two **efferent** nerve fibers, whose job is to convey messages from the brain to the hair cells. When fluid moves in the cochlea, the hair cells inside the organ of Corti start to bend in response to the vibrations that the fluid influx produces. The small movements then cause excitation of the hair cells and of the afferent axons. The sound stimulus is translated into electrical signals that are sent to the auditory brainstem and auditory cortex of the brain.

Taste

Humans can detect five basic tastes with gustatory (taste nerve) cells: sweet, salty, sour, bitter, and umami. The human tongue has small projections, called **papillae**, that contain most of the taste receptor cells, or taste buds. Each papilla has one or more clusters of 50 to 150 taste buds. In addition to the taste buds, the papillae also contain pain receptors, which can sense spice for example, and touch receptors.

Taste buds are specific for one of the five taste sensations and are activated through different mechanisms. Below are descriptions of how each taste is sensed by the brain.

Salty

Salt-sensing taste buds are activated when sodium ions are transported across the membrane of the taste bud through sodium ion channels. The taste buds get partially depolarized, causing a release of neurotransmitters. This stimulates afferent neurons, which relay the stimulation information to the brain.

Sour

Sour tastes are sensed when sour foods or drinks release a hydrogen ion, which blocks the potassium channels of the taste bud membranes. The build-up of potassium in the cell leads to depolarization, neurotransmitter release, and stimulation information gets sent to the brain.

Sweet

The taste buds that sense sweetness have a more complicated stimulation pathway than those of the salty and sour taste buds. When sweet molecules bind to the receptors on their taste buds, a conformational change occurs in the molecule, which then activates a G-protein called **gustducin.** Several other proteins are activated along the pathway, which eventually leads to a blockage of potassium ion channels and an opening of a calcium ion channel. The influx of calcium to the cell causes a greater depolarization of the cell, release of neurotransmitters, and afferent neurons transmit the stimulation information to the brain.

Bitter

The bitter taste sensation has an even more complex pathway than that of sweetness. Bitterness is thought to be the most sensitive of the tastes and is often perceived as sharp and unpleasant. In a similar pathway to the sweet taste, taste receptors are coupled to the G-protein gustducin. When a bitter substance is sensed, the gustducin breaks apart. Potassium ion channels are closed, calcium ion channels are opened, and the taste cell is depolarized. Neurotransmitters are released, and afferent neurons transmit stimulation information to the brain.

Umami

The taste of umami, which may be described as a meaty or savory flavor, was only relatively recently recognized as a separate taste. The receptors for umami react to glutamates and nucleotides, which are both found abundantly in meats and fermented foods. The fermenting process for many foods frees glutamic acid from proteins which creates ionic bonds with various cations to form different glutamates. Like with sweet and bitter flavors, when umami receptors bind to umami molecules, the receptors activate G proteins which are part of the pathway to sense umami via gustatory nerves.

Smell

Olfactory Cells and Chemoreceptors

The dorsal portion of the nasal cavities is lined with an **olfactory epithelium**. This epithelium contains the receptor neurons that sense smell. If the olfactory epithelium is ever damaged, it has the capability to regenerate itself, including replacement of the receptor neurons. The chemical nature of odors is important for distinguishing between them because odors bind to olfactory receptors that are specific for a certain functional group of the odorant.

Pheromones

In addition to the main olfactory epithelium, the olfactory system has a **vomeronasal organ (VNO)**. Both organs are responsible for detecting pheromones, which are secreted chemicals that trigger a social reaction from members of the same species.

Olfactory Pathways in the Brain

The axons of the olfactory nerves terminate at the anterior end of the brain in a structure called the **olfactory bulb**. The olfactory bulb is organized into **glomeruli**, which are spherically-shaped neural circuits. The output from the bulb goes to the prepyriform area, the amygdala, and the hypothalamus within the brain for information processing.

Touch

The **special senses** include vision, hearing and balance, smell, and taste. They are distinguished from general senses in that special senses have special somatic afferents and special visceral afferents, both a type of nerve fiber relaying information to the CNS, as well as specialized organs devoted to their function. Touch is the other sense that is typically discussed, but unlike the special senses, it relays information to the CNS from all over the body and not just one particular organ; **skin**, the largest organ of the body, is the largest contributor to tactile information, but touch receptors also include **mechanoreceptors** (for touch, pressure, and sound), **nociceptors** (for pain), and **thermoreceptors** (for heat). Tactile messages are carried via general somatic afferents and general visceral afferents. Various touch receptors exist in the body such as the following:

- Pacinian corpuscles: detect rapid vibration in the skin and fascia
- Meissner's corpuscles: respond to light touch and slower vibrations
- Merkel's discs: respond to sustained pressure
- Ruffini endings: detect deep touch and tension in the skin and fascia

Somatosensation

Somatosensation is the reception and interpretation of sensory information that comes from specialized organs in the joints, ligaments, muscles, and skin. The somatosensory system consists of nerve cells, or sensory receptors, that respond to changes in these organs, including pressure, texture, temperature, and pain. Signals are sent along a chain of nerve cells to the spinal cord and then to the brain for information processing. Nociceptors are sensory receptors that detect pain in a range from acute and tolerable to chronic and intolerable. Nociceptors are divided into mechanosensitive nociceptors (mechanical force), mechanothermal nociceptors (mechanical and thermal stimuli), and polymodal nociceptors (chemical, mechanical, and thermal stimuli). Muscles and joints contain mostly **proprioceptors**, which detect joint position and movement, as well as the direction and velocity of the movement.

Kinesthetic Sense

Kinesthetic sense is the sensation of movement and orientation. This sense is composed of information that comes from the sensory receptors in the inner ear regarding motion and orientation as well as in the stretch receptors that are in the muscles and ligaments, which provide information about stance. When the brain receives information regarding these movements, it can help to control and coordinate the body's actions, such as simultaneous walking and talking.

Vestibular Sense

Vestibular sense includes the sense of balance and spatial orientation. Combining these two things allows for the coordination of movement and balance. The receptors for the vestibular system are also found within the inner ear. This system allows the brain to understand how the body is moving and accelerating at each moment.

Perception

Perception is the interpretation of sensory information in order to understand the environment. It begins with an object stimulating one or more of the sensory organs in the body. For example, light stimulates the retina in the eye and odor molecules stimulate the receptors in the nasal cavity. In a process called transduction, this stimulation information is transformed into neural activity. These neural signals are then transmitted to the brain and processed there. The brain then creates a memory of this stimulus. When an unfamiliar object is encountered, the brain tries to collect as much information about the object as possible. When a familiar object is encountered again, the brain uses the senses to confirm that the object is indeed the familiar one.

Bottom-up and top-down processing are two different methods of information processing. Sensory input is considered bottom-up processing while top-down processing involves the organization of information from many different sources and is considered a more complex process. Bottom-up processing can be described as a progression from individual elements to a complete picture. A stimulus is seen clearly, and the brain can make sense of the object using only the senses. Top-down processing involves the receipt of vague sensory information followed by the resolution of it using internal hypotheses and expectation interactions. The brain uses more than just the sensory areas to figure out what the stimulus is.

Sensory organs help resolve different facets about an object. Depth perception is how a person judges their distance from an object. Each eye has a slightly different view on the same object, which can help distinguish where an object is located and what it fully looks like. The relative size of two objects can be distinguished by the differently sized images that are projected onto the retina. **Relative motion** can be determined by detecting that objects closer than the visual point of focus are moving in the opposite direction of the viewer's moving head and vice versa. **Perceptual constancy** is the idea that objects are stable and unchanging despite changes in sensory stimulation. The brain can identify familiar objects at any distance, from any angle, and with any illumination. Shape, color, and brightness are all perceived the same as they were originally. For example, a woman standing one hundred feet away appears small, but the brain knows what her actual height is and processes it as such.

Practice Quiz

1. Which statement about white blood cells is true?
   a. B cells are responsible for antibody production.
   b. White blood cells are made in the white/yellow cartilage before they enter the bloodstream.
   c. Platelets, a special class of white blood cell, function to clot blood and stop bleeding.
   d. The majority of white blood cells only activate during the age of puberty, which explains why children and the elderly are particularly susceptible to disease.

2. Which locations in the digestive system are sites of chemical digestion?

   I. Mouth
   II. Stomach
   III. Small Intestine

   a. II only
   b. III only
   c. II and III only
   d. I, II, and III

3. Which of the following are functions of the urinary system?
   - I. Synthesizing calcitriol and secreting erythropoietin
   - II. Regulating the concentrations of sodium, potassium, chloride, calcium, and other ions
   - III. Reabsorbing or secreting hydrogen ions and bicarbonate
   - IV. Detecting reductions in blood volume and pressure

   a. I, II, and III
   b. II and III
   c. II, III, and IV
   d. I, II, III, and IV

4. When de-oxygenated blood enters the heart, which chamber does it enter first?
   a. Right atrium
   b. Left atrium
   c. Right ventricle
   d. Left ventricle

5. What is the purpose of sodium bicarbonate when released into the lumen of the small intestine?
   a. It works to chemically digest fats in the chyme.
   b. It decreases the pH of the chyme so as to prevent harm to the intestine.
   c. It works to chemically digest proteins in the chyme.
   d. It increases the pH of the chyme so as to prevent harm to the intestine.

See answers on the next page.

Answer Explanations

1. A: When activated, B cells create antibodies against specific antigens. White blood cells are generated in the red bone marrow, not in cartilage. Platelets are not a type of white blood cell and are typically cell fragments produced by megakaryocytes. White blood cells are active throughout nearly all of one's life and have not been shown to specially activate or deactivate because of life events like puberty or menopause.

2. D: Mechanical digestion is physical digestion of food by tearing it into smaller pieces using force. This occurs in the stomach and mouth. Chemical digestion involves chemically changing the food and breaking it down into small organic compounds that can be utilized by the cell to build molecules. The salivary glands in the mouth secrete amylase that breaks down starch, which begins chemical digestion. The stomach contains enzymes such as pepsinogen/pepsin and gastric lipase which chemically digest protein and fats, respectively. The small intestine continues to digest protein using the enzymes trypsin and chymotrypsin. It also digests fats with the help of bile from the liver and lipase from the pancreas. These organs act as exocrine glands because they secrete substances through a duct. Carbohydrates are digested in the small intestine with the help of pancreatic amylase, gut bacterial flora and fauna, and brush border enzymes like lactose. Brush border enzymes are contained in the towel-like microvilli in the small intestine that soak up nutrients.

3. D: The urinary system has many functions, the primary of which is removing waste products and balancing water and electrolyte concentrations in the blood. It also plays a key role in regulating ion concentrations, such as sodium, potassium, chloride, and calcium, in the filtrate. The urinary system helps maintain blood pH by reabsorbing or secreting hydrogen ions and bicarbonate as necessary. Certain kidney cells can detect reductions in blood volume and pressure and then can secrete renin to activate a hormone that causes increased reabsorption of sodium ions and water. This serves to raise blood volume and pressure. Kidney cells secrete erythropoietin under hypoxic conditions to stimulate red blood cell production. They also synthesize calcitriol, a hormone derivative of vitamin D3, which aids in calcium ion absorption by the intestinal epithelium.

4. A: Carbon dioxide-rich blood is delivered from systemic circulation to the right atrium. It is pumped into the right ventricle. The tricuspid valve prevents backflow between the two chambers. From there, the pulmonary artery takes blood to the lungs where diffusion causes gas exchange. Then, oxygenated blood returns to the left atrium before getting pumped into the left ventricle. The mitral valve prevents the backflow of blood from the left ventricle to the atrium. Finally, blood is ejected from the left ventricle through the aorta to enter systemic circulation.

5. D: Sodium bicarbonate, a very effective base, functions chiefly to increase the pH of the chyme. Chyme leaving the stomach has a very low pH due to the high amounts of acid that are used to digest and break down food. If this is not neutralized, the walls of the small intestine will be damaged and may form ulcers. Sodium bicarbonate is produced by the pancreas and released in response to pyloric stimulation so that it can neutralize the acid. It has little to no digestive effect.

Practice Test #1

Reading Comprehension

The next six questions are based on the following passage:

When researchers and engineers undertake a large-scale scientific project, they may end up making discoveries and developing technologies that have far wider uses than originally intended. This is especially true at NASA, one of the most influential and innovative scientific organizations in America. NASA spinoff technology refers to innovations originally developed for NASA space projects that are now used in a wide range of different commercial fields. Many consumers are unaware that products they are buying are based on NASA research! Spinoff technology proves that it is worthwhile to invest in scientific research because it could enrich people's lives in unexpected ways.

The first spinoff technology worth mentioning is baby food. In space, where astronauts have limited access to fresh food and fewer options about their daily meals, malnutrition is a serious concern. Consequently, NASA researchers were looking for ways to enhance the nutritional value of astronauts' food. Scientists found that a certain type of algae could be added to food to improve the food's neurological benefits. When experts in the commercial food industry learned of this algae's potential to boost brain health, they were quick to begin their own research. The nutritional substance from algae was developed into a product called life's DHA, which can be found in over 90% of infant food sold in America.

Another intriguing example of a spinoff technology can be found in fashion. People who are always dropping their sunglasses may have invested in a pair of sunglasses with scratch-resistant lenses, which are made of glass that is impossible to scratch, even when dropped on an abrasive surface. This innovation is incredibly advantageous for people who are clumsy, but most shoppers don't know that this technology was originally developed by NASA. Scientists first created scratch-resistant glass to help protect costly and crucial equipment from getting scratched in space, especially the helmet visors in space suits. However, sunglasses companies later realized that this technology could be profitable for their products, and they licensed the technology from NASA.

1. What is the main purpose of this article?
    a. To advise consumers to do more research before making a purchase
    b. To persuade readers to support NASA's research
    c. To tell a narrative about the history of space technology
    d. To define and describe instances of spinoff technology

2. What is the organizational structure of this article?
    a. A general definition followed by more specific examples
    b. A general opinion followed by supporting evidence
    c. An important moment in history followed by chronological details
    d. A popular misconception followed by counterevidence

3. Why did NASA scientists research algae?
    a. They already knew algae was healthy for babies.
    b. They were interested in how to grow food in space.
    c. They were looking for ways to add health benefits to food.
    d. They hoped to use it to protect expensive research equipment.

4. What does the word *neurological* mean in the second paragraph?
    a. Related to the body
    b. Related to the brain
    c. Related to vitamins
    d. Related to technology

5. Why does the author mention space suit helmets?
    a. To give an example of astronaut fashion
    b. To explain where sunglasses got their shape from
    c. To explain how astronauts protect their eyes
    d. To give an example of valuable space equipment

6. Which statement would the author probably NOT agree with?
    a. Consumers don't always know the history of the products they are buying.
    b. Sometimes new innovations have unexpected applications.
    c. It is difficult to make money from scientific research.
    d. Space equipment is often very expensive.

The next seven questions are based on the following passage:

> People who argue that William Shakespeare is not responsible for the plays attributed to his name are known as anti-Stratfordians (from the name of Shakespeare's birthplace, Stratford-upon-Avon). The most common anti-Stratfordian claim is that William Shakespeare simply was not educated enough or from a high enough social class to have written plays overflowing with references to such a wide range of subjects, like history, the classics, religion, and international culture. William Shakespeare was the son of a glove-maker, he only had a basic grade-school education, and he never set foot outside of England—so how could he have produced plays of such sophistication and imagination? How could he have written in such detail about historical figures and events, or about different cultures and locations around Europe? According to anti-Stratfordians, the depth of knowledge contained in Shakespeare's plays suggests a well-traveled writer from a wealthy background with a university education, not a countryside writer like Shakespeare. But in fact, there is not much substance to such speculation, and most anti-Stratfordian arguments can be refuted with a little background about Shakespeare's time and upbringing.
>
> First of all, those who doubt Shakespeare's authorship often point to his common birth and brief education as stumbling blocks to his writerly genius. Although it is true that Shakespeare did not come from a noble class, his father was a very *successful* glove-maker, and his mother was from a very wealthy land-owning family—so while Shakespeare may have had a country upbringing, he was certainly from a well-off family and would have been educated accordingly. Also, even though he did not attend university, grade-school education in Shakespeare's time was actually quite rigorous and

exposed students to classic drama through writers like Seneca and Ovid. It is not unreasonable to believe that Shakespeare received a very solid foundation in poetry and literature from his early schooling.

Next, anti-Stratfordians tend to question how Shakespeare could write so extensively about countries and cultures he had never visited before. For instance, several of his most famous works, like *Romeo and Juliet* and *The Merchant of Venice*, were set in Italy, which is located on the opposite side of Europe from England. But again, this criticism does not hold up under scrutiny. For one thing, Shakespeare was living in London, a bustling metropolis of international trade, the most populous city in England, and a political and cultural hub of Europe. In the daily crowds of people, Shakespeare would certainly have been able to meet travelers from other countries and hear firsthand accounts of life in their home country. And, in addition to the influx of information from world travelers, this was also the age of the printing press. This jump in technology made it possible to print and circulate books much more easily than in the past. This also facilitated a freer flow of information across different countries, allowing people to read about life and ideas from all over Europe. One needn't travel the continent in order to learn and write about its different cultures.

7. What is the main purpose of this article?
   a. To explain two sides of an argument and allow readers to choose which side they agree with
   b. To encourage readers to be skeptical about the authorship of famous poems and plays
   c. To give historical background on an important literary figure
   d. To criticize a theory by presenting counterevidence

8. Which sentence contains the author's thesis?
   a. People who argue that William Shakespeare is not responsible for the plays attributed to his name are known as anti-Stratfordians.
   b. But in fact, there is not much substance to such speculation, and most anti-Stratfordian arguments can be refuted with a little background about Shakespeare's time and upbringing.
   c. It is not unreasonable to believe that Shakespeare received a very solid foundation in poetry and literature from his early schooling.
   d. Next, anti-Stratfordians tend to question how Shakespeare could write so extensively about countries and cultures he had never visited before.

9. How does the author respond to the claim that Shakespeare was not well-educated because he did not attend university?
   a. By insisting upon Shakespeare's natural genius
   b. By explaining grade-school curriculum in Shakespeare's time
   c. By comparing Shakespeare with other uneducated writers of his time
   d. By pointing out that Shakespeare's wealthy parents probably paid for private tutors

10. What does the word "bustling" in the third paragraph most nearly mean?
   a. Busy
   b. Foreign
   c. Expensive
   d. Undeveloped

11. What can be inferred from the article?
    a. Shakespeare's peers were jealous of his success and wanted to attack his reputation.
    b. Until recently, classic drama was only taught in universities.
    c. International travel was extremely rare in Shakespeare's time.
    d. In Shakespeare's time, glove-makers were not part of the upper class.

12. Why does the author mention *Romeo and Juliet*?
    a. It is Shakespeare's most famous play.
    b. It was inspired by Shakespeare's trip to Italy.
    c. It is an example of a play set outside of England.
    d. It was unpopular when Shakespeare first wrote it.

13. Which statement would the author probably agree with?
    a. It is possible to learn things from reading rather than from firsthand experience.
    b. If you want to be truly cultured, you need to travel the world.
    c. People never become successful without a university education.
    d. All of the world's great art comes from Italy.

Questions 14-17 are based on the following passage:

> Four score and seven years ago our fathers brought forth on this continent, a new nation, conceived in Liberty, and dedicated to the proposition that all men are created equal.
>
> Now we are engaged in a great civil war, testing whether that nation, or any nation so conceived and so dedicated, can long endure. We are met on a great battle-field of that war. We have come to dedicate a portion of that field, as a final resting place for those who here gave their lives that that nation might live. It is altogether fitting and proper that we should do this.
>
> But, in a larger sense, we cannot dedicate — we cannot consecrate that we cannot hallow — this ground. The brave men, living and dead, who struggled here, have consecrated it, far above our poor power to add or detract. The world will little note, nor long remember what we say here, but it can never forget what they did here. It is for us the living, rather, to be dedicated here to the unfinished work which they who fought here have thus far so nobly advanced. It is rather for us to be here dedicated to the great task remaining before us — that from these honored dead we take increased devotion to that cause for which they gave the last full measure of devotion — that we here highly resolve that these dead shall not have died in vain - that this nation, under God, shall have a new birth of freedom — and that government of the people, by the people, for the people, shall not perish from the earth.
>
> Address by Abraham Lincoln, delivered at the dedication of the cemetery at Gettysburg,1863

14. The best description for the phrase "Four score and seven years ago" is:
    a. A unit of measurement
    b. A period of time
    c. A literary movement
    d. A statement of political reform

15. Which war is Abraham Lincoln referring to in the following passage?

> Now we are engaged in a great civil war, testing whether that nation, or any nation so conceived and so dedicated, can long endure.

a. World War I
b. The War of Spanish Succession
c. World War II
d. The American Civil War

16. What message is the speaker trying to convey through this address?
a. The audience should honor the dead by completing the goal they died to achieve.
b. The audience should honor the dead by establishing an annual memorial service.
c. The audience should form a militia that would overturn the current political structure.
d. The audience should forget the lives that were lost and discredit the soldiers.

17. What is the effect of Lincoln's statement in the following passage? "But, in a larger sense, we cannot dedicate — we cannot consecrate that we cannot hallow — this ground. The brave men, living and dead, who struggled here, have consecrated it, far above our poor power to add or detract."
a. His comparison emphasizes the great sacrifice of the soldiers who fought in the war.
b. His comparison serves as a reminder of the inadequacies of his audience.
c. His comparison serves as a catalyst for guilt and shame among audience members.
d. His comparison suggests that the dedication ceremony was inappropriate.

Questions 18-22 are based on the following passage:

> As long ago as 1860 it was the proper thing to be born at home. At present, so I am told, the high gods of medicine have decreed that the first cries of the young shall be uttered upon the anesthetic air of a hospital, preferably a fashionable one. So young Mr. and Mrs. Roger Button were fifty years ahead of style when they decided, one day in the summer of 1860, that their first baby should be born in a hospital. Whether this anachronism had any bearing upon the astonishing history I am about to set down will never be known.
>
> I shall tell you what occurred, and let you judge for yourself.
>
> The Roger Buttons held an enviable position, both social and financial, in ante-bellum Baltimore. They were related to the This Family and the That Family, which, as every Southerner knew, entitled them to membership in that enormous peerage which largely populated the Confederacy. This was their first experience with the charming old custom of having babies—Mr. Button was naturally nervous. He hoped it would be a boy so that he could be sent to Yale College in Connecticut, at which institution Mr. Button himself had been known for four years by the somewhat obvious nickname of "Cuff."
>
> On the September morning consecrated to the enormous event he arose nervously at six o'clock, dressed himself, adjusted an impeccable stock, and hurried forth through the streets of Baltimore to the hospital, to determine whether the darkness of the night had borne in new life upon its bosom.

When he was approximately a hundred yards from the Maryland Private Hospital for Ladies and Gentlemen he saw Doctor Keene, the family physician, descending the front steps, rubbing his hands together with a washing movement—as all doctors are required to do by the unwritten ethics of their profession.

Mr. Roger Button, the president of Roger Button & Co., Wholesale Hardware, began to run toward Doctor Keene with much less dignity than was expected from a Southern gentleman of that picturesque period. "Doctor Keene!" he called. "Oh, Doctor Keene!"

The doctor heard him, faced around, and stood waiting, a curious expression settling on his harsh, medicinal face as Mr. Button drew near.

"What happened?" demanded Mr. Button, as he came up in a gasping rush. "What was it? How is she? A boy? Who is it? What—"

"Talk sense!" said Doctor Keene sharply. He appeared somewhat irritated.

"Is the child born?" begged Mr. Button.

Doctor Keene frowned. "Why, yes, I suppose so—after a fashion." Again he threw a curious glance at Mr. Button.

The Curious Case of Benjamin Button, F. S. Fitzgerald, 1922

18. What major event is about to happen in this story?
    a. Mr. Button is about to go to a funeral.
    b. Mr. Button's wife is about to have a baby.
    c. Mr. Button is getting ready to go to the doctor's office.
    d. Mr. Button is about to go shopping for new clothes.

19. What kind of tone does the above passage have?
    a. Nervous and excited
    b. Sad and angry
    c. Shameful and confused
    d. Grateful and joyous

20. What is the meaning of the word "consecrated" in paragraph 4?
    a. Numbed
    b. Chained
    c. Dedicated
    d. Moved

21. What does the author mean to do by adding the following description?

    rubbing his hands together with a washing movement—as all doctors are required to do by the unwritten ethics of their profession.

    a. Suggest that Mr. Button is tired of the doctor
    b. Try to explain the details of the doctor's profession
    c. Hint to readers that the doctor is an unethical man
    d. Give readers a visual picture of what the doctor is doing

22. Which of the following best describes the development of this passage?
    a. It starts in the middle of a narrative in order to transition smoothly to a conclusion.
    b. It is a chronological narrative from beginning to end.
    c. The sequence of events is backwards—we go from future events to past events.
    d. It introduces the setting of the story and its characters.

Writing

The next six questions are based on the following passage:

> [1]While all dogs descend through gray wolves, it's easy to notice that dog breeds come in a variety of shapes and sizes. [2] With such a drastic range of traits appearances and body types, dogs are one of the most variable and adaptable species on the planet. [3] But why are there so many differences. [4]The answer is that humans have actually played a major role in altering the biology of dogs. [5]This was done through a process called selective breeding.
>
> [6]Selective breeding is the process in which animals with desired traits are bred to produce offspring that share the same traits and it is also known as artificial selection. [7]In natural evolution, animals must adopt to their environments to increase their chance of survival. [8]Over time, certain traits develop in animals that enable them to thrive in these environments. [9] The animals that have more of these traits, or better versions of these traits, gain an advantage over others of their species. [10]Therefore, the animal's chances to mate are increased, and these useful genes are passed into their offspring. [11]With dog breeding, humans select traits that are desired and encourage more of these desired traits in other dogs by breeding dogs that already have them.

1. Which sentence in the first paragraph uses an incorrect preposition?
    a. Sentence 1
    b. Sentence 2
    c. Sentence 4
    d. Sentence 5

2. Which sentence in the passage is a run-on sentence?
    a. Sentence 2
    b. Sentence 6
    c. Sentence 9
    d. Sentence 11

3. Which sentence is missing an Oxford comma?
    a. Sentence 2
    b. Sentence 9
    c. Sentence 10
    d. Sentence 11

4. Which word in the second paragraph is incorrect?
   a. Offspring
   b. Adopt
   c. Traits
   d. Species

5. Which sentence has an end punctuation error?
   a. Sentence 2
   b. Sentence 3
   c. Sentence 6
   d. Sentence 10

6. Which sentence in the second paragraph uses the incorrect preposition?
   a. Sentence 6
   b. Sentence 9
   c. Sentence 10
   d. Sentence 11

The next seven questions are based on the following passage:

> [1]As the adage goes knowledge is power. [2]Those who are smart and understand the world as it is are the most fit to lead. [3]Intelligence doesn't necessarily require a deep understanding of complex scientific principles. [4]Rather, having the basic knowledge of how the world works, particularly how people go about gaining what they need to survive and thrive, are more important.
>
> [5]Any leadership position, whether on the job or informally, tends to be fraught with politics. [6]Smart leaders will engage in critical thinking allowing them to discern ulterior motives and identify propaganda. [7]Besides catching negative intentions, these practice will serve to highlight the positives in group interactions. [8]Gaining insights into different viewpoints will make leaders more receptive for constructive criticism and ideas from unexpected sources. [9]As with many aspects of being a good and well-rounded person, the seeds for this trait are sown in pre-school. [10]Besides facts and figures, students need to be taught critical thinking skills to survive in a world flooded with subliminal messages and scams. [11]Sadly, our current society is plaguing by many inconvenient truths that are attacked as lies. [12]Wise leaders should recognize when someone is trying to save the world or merely push a political agenda.

7. Which sentence in the first paragraph contains a subject-verb agreement error?
   a. Sentence 1
   b. Sentence 2
   c. Sentence 3
   d. Sentence 4

8. Which of the following is a punctuation error in the first paragraph?
   a. Sentence 2 should have ended in an exclamation point.
   b. Sentence 4 needed a semicolon instead of a comma after the word *works*.
   c. Sentence 3 has an apostrophe in the wrong place.
   d. Sentence 1 is missing quotation marks.

9. Which sentence in the first paragraph is missing a necessary comma?
    a. Sentence 1
    b. Sentence 2
    c. Sentence 3
    d. Sentence 4

10. Which sentence contains an error involving a gerund?
    a. Sentence 7
    b. Sentence 8
    c. Sentence 11
    d. Sentence 12

11. Which sentence in the second paragraph is missing a necessary comma?
    a. Sentence 6
    b. Sentence 8
    c. Sentence 9
    d. Sentence 10

12. Which sentence in the second paragraph has an error in numerical agreement between a demonstrative pronoun and a noun?
    a. Sentence 6
    b. Sentence 7
    c. Sentence 9
    d. Sentence 11

13. Which sentence in the second paragraph uses an incorrect preposition?
    a. Sentence 8
    b. Sentence 9
    c. Sentence 10
    d. Sentence 11

Questions 14-21 are based on the following passage:

> [1]The knowledge of an aircraft engineer is acquitted through years of education, and special licenses are often required. [2]Ideally, an individual will begin their preparation for the profession in high school by taking chemistry physics trigonometry and calculus. [3]High school students often enjoy playing sports, spending time with friends, and watch TV. [4]Such curricula will aid in ones pursuit of a bachelor's degree in aircraft engineering, which requires several physical and life sciences, mathematics, and design courses.
>
> [5]Some of universities provide internship or apprenticeship opportunities for the students enrolled in aircraft engineering programs. [6]A bachelor's in aircraft engineering is commonly accompanied by a master's degree in advanced engineering or business administration. [7]Such advanced degrees enable an individual to position himself or herself for executive, faculty, and/or research opportunities. [8]These advanced offices oftentimes require a Professional Engineering (PE) license; which can be obtained through additional college courses, professional experience, and acceptable scores on the Fundamentals of Engineering (FE) and Professional Engineering (PE) standardized assessments.

> [9]Once the job begins, this lines of work requires critical thinking, business skills, problem solving, and creativity. [10]This level of expertise requires aircraft engineers to apply mathematical equation and scientific processes to aeronautical and aerospace issues or inventions. [11]For example, aircraft engineers may test, design, and construct flying vessels such as airplanes, space shuttles, and missile weapons. [12]As a result, aircraft engineers are compensated with generous salaries, the job outlook is good.

14. Which sentence in the first paragraph is missing commas?
    a. Sentence 1
    b. Sentence 2
    c. Sentence 3
    d. Sentence 4

15. Which sentence has an error regarding an apostrophe?
    a. Sentence 1
    b. Sentence 4
    c. Sentence 6
    d. Sentence 8

16. Which of the following is an error in the second paragraph?
    a. *Bachelor's* and *master's* in Sentence 6 do not need apostrophes
    b. Sentence 7 is missing a colon after *for*
    c. Sentence 8 has a semicolon instead of a comma
    d. Sentence 8 has capitalized words that do not need to be capitalized

17. Which sentence has an extra preposition that does not belong?
    a. Sentence 4
    b. Sentence 5
    c. Sentence 9
    d. Sentence 11

18. Which sentence is unrelated to the passage and should be removed?
    a. Sentence 2
    b. Sentence 3
    c. Sentence 6
    d. Sentence 9

19. Which sentence has an agreement error?
    a. Sentence 4
    b. Sentence 7
    c. Sentence 9
    d. Sentence 11

20. Which sentence is a run-on?
    a. Sentence 4
    b. Sentence 8
    c. Sentence 10
    d. Sentence 12

21. Which word in context is incorrect?
    a. Acquitted
    b. Curricula
    c. Apprenticeship
    d. Obtained

Mathematics

1. What is 3 out of 8 expressed as a percent?
    a. 37.5%
    b. 37%
    c. 26.7%
    d. 2.67%

2. What is 39% of 164?
    a. 63.96
    b. 23.78
    c. 6,396
    d. 2.38

3. 32 is 25% of what number?
    a. 64
    b. 128
    c. 12.65
    d. 8

4. Convert $\frac{5}{8}$ to a decimal, rounding to the nearest hundredth.
    a. 0.62
    b. 1.05
    c. 0.63
    d. 1.60

5. Change $3\frac{3}{5}$ to a decimal.
    a. 3.6
    b. 4.67
    c. 5.3
    d. 0.28

6. Change 0.56 to a fraction.
    a. $\frac{5.6}{100}$
    b. $\frac{14}{25}$
    c. $\frac{56}{1,000}$
    d. $\frac{56}{10}$

7. Change 9.3 to a fraction or a mixed number.
   a. $9\frac{3}{7}$
   b. $\frac{903}{1,000}$
   c. $\frac{9.03}{100}$
   d. $9\frac{3}{10}$

8. The hospital has a nurse-to-patient ratio of $1:25$. If a maximum of 325 patients may be admitted at a time, how many nurses are there?
   a. 13 nurses
   b. 25 nurses
   c. 325 nurses
   d. 12 nurses

9. A hospital has a bed-to-room ratio of $2:1$. If there are 145 rooms, how many beds are there?
   a. 145 beds
   b. 2 beds
   c. 90 beds
   d. 290 beds

10. Solve for x. $\frac{2x}{5} - 1 = 59$.
   a. 60
   b. 145
   c. 150
   d. 115

11. Store-brand coffee beans cost \$1.23 per pound. A local coffee bean roaster charges \$1.98 per $1\frac{1}{2}$ pounds. How much more would 5 pounds from the local roaster cost than 5 pounds of the store-brand?
   a. \$0.55
   b. \$1.55
   c. \$1.45
   d. \$0.45

12. Paint Inc. charges \$2,000 for painting the first 1,800 feet of trim on a house and an additional \$1.00 per foot for each foot beyond that. How much would it cost to paint a house with 3,125 feet of trim?
   a. \$3,125
   b. \$2,000
   c. \$5,125
   d. \$3,325

13. Which of the following values is the largest?
   a. 0.45
   b. 0.096
   c. 0.3
   d. 0.313

14. Which of the following is NOT a way to write 40% of N?
   a. $(0.4)N$
   b. $\frac{2}{5}N$
   c. $40N$
   d. $\frac{4}{10}N$

15. Four people split a bill. The first person pays for $\frac{1}{5}$, the second person pays for $\frac{1}{4}$, and the third person pays for $\frac{1}{3}$. What fraction of the bill does the fourth person pay?
   a. $\frac{13}{60}$
   b. $\frac{47}{60}$
   c. $\frac{1}{4}$
   d. $\frac{4}{15}$

16. A closet is filled with red, blue, and green shirts. If $\frac{1}{3}$ of the shirts are green and $\frac{2}{5}$ are red, what fraction of the shirts are blue?
   a. $\frac{4}{15}$
   b. $\frac{1}{5}$
   c. $\frac{7}{15}$
   d. $\frac{1}{2}$

17. Shawna buys $2\frac{1}{2}$ gallons of paint. If she uses $\frac{1}{3}$ of it on the first day, how much does she have left?
   a. $1\frac{5}{6}$ gallons
   b. $1\frac{1}{2}$ gallons
   c. $1\frac{2}{3}$ gallons
   d. 2 gallons

18. How would $\frac{4}{5}$ be written as a percent?
   a. 40%
   b. 125%
   c. 90%
   d. 80%

19. At the beginning of the day, Xavier has 20 apples. At lunch, he meets his sister Emma and gives her half of his apples. After lunch, he stops by his neighbor Jim's house and gives him six of his apples. He then uses $\frac{3}{4}$ of his remaining apples to make an apple pie for dessert at dinner. At the end of the day, how many apples does Xavier have left?
   a. 4
   b. 6
   c. 2
   d. 1

20. If $4x - 3 = 5$, what is the value of x?
   a. 1
   b. 2
   c. 3
   d. 4

21. On Monday, Robert mopped the floor in 4 hours. On Tuesday, he did it in 3 hours. If on Monday, his average rate of mopping was p sq. ft. per hour, what was his average rate on Tuesday?
   a. $\frac{4p}{3}$ sq. ft. per hour
   b. $\frac{3}{4}p$ sq. ft. per hour
   c. $\frac{5}{4}p$ sq. ft. per hour
   d. $p + 1$ sq. ft. per hour

22. Alan currently weighs 200 pounds, but he wants to lose weight to get down to 175 pounds. What is this difference in kilograms? (1 pound is approximately equal to 0.45 kilograms.)
   a. 9 kg
   b. 11.25 kg
   c. 78.75 kg
   d. 7.5 kg

23. An emergency department had 252 patients last week. This week, that number increased to 378. Express this increase as a percentage.
   a. 26%
   b. 50%
   c. 35%
   d. 12%

24. After a 20% sale discount, Frank purchased a new refrigerator for $850. How much money did he save off of the original price?
   a. $170
   b. $212.50
   c. $105.75
   d. $200

25. A construction company is building a new housing development with the property of each house measuring 30 feet wide. If the length of the street is zoned off at 345 feet, how many houses can be built on the street?

a. 11 houses
b. 115 houses
c. 11.5 houses
d. 12 houses

26. Mo needs to buy enough material to cover the walls around the stage for a theater performance. If he needs 79 feet of wall covering, what is the minimum number of yards of material he should purchase if the material is sold only by whole yards?

a. 23 yards
b. 25 yards
c. 26 yards
d. 27 yards

27. You measure the width of your door to be 36 inches. The true width of the door is 35.75 inches. What is the relative error in your measurement?

a. 0.7%
b. 0.007%
c. 0.99%
d. 0.1%

28. A couple buys a house for $150,000. They sell it for $165,000. By what percentage did the house's value increase?

a. 10%
b. 13%
c. 15%
d. 17%

Science

1. Which of the following describes a reflex arc?

a. The storage and recall of memory
b. The maintenance of visual and auditory acuity
c. The autoregulation of heart rate and blood pressure
d. A stimulus and response controlled by the spinal cord

2. Which of the following structures acts like a funnel by delivering the urine from the millions of collecting tubules to the ureters?

a. The renal pelvis
b. The renal cortex
c. The renal medulla
d. Bowman's capsule

3. Which of the following are responsible for the exchange of nutrients, hormones, oxygen, fluids, and electrolytes between blood and the interstitial fluid of body tissues?
   a. Arterioles
   b. Venules
   c. Capillaries
   d. Hemoglobin

4. Which of the following is NOT a major function of the respiratory system in humans?
   a. It provides a large surface area for gas exchange of oxygen and carbon dioxide.
   b. It helps regulate the blood's pH.
   c. It helps cushion the heart against jarring motions.
   d. It is responsible for vocalization.

5. Which of the following is NOT a function of the forebrain?
   a. To regulate blood pressure and heart rate
   b. To perceive and interpret emotional responses like fear and anger
   c. To perceive and interpret visual input from the eyes
   d. To integrate voluntary movement

6. A patient's body is not properly filtering blood. Which of the following body parts is most likely malfunctioning?
   a. Medulla
   b. Heart
   c. Nephrons
   d. Renal cortex

7. A cluster of capillaries that functions as the main filter of the blood entering the kidney is known as which of the following?
   a. The Bowman's capsule
   b. The loop of Henle
   c. The glomerulus
   d. The nephron

8. Which of the following correctly identifies a difference between the primary and secondary immune responses?
   a. In the secondary response, macrophages migrate to the lymph nodes to present the foreign microorganism to helper T lymphocytes.
   b. The humoral immunity that characterizes the primary response is coordinated by T lymphocytes.
   c. The primary response is quicker and more powerful than the secondary response.
   d. Suppressor T cells activate in the secondary response to prevent an overactive immune response.

9. Which of the following functions corresponds to the parasympathetic nervous system?
   a. It stimulates the fight-or-flight response.
   b. It increases heart rate.
   c. It stimulates digestion.
   d. It increases bronchiole dilation.

10. What is the order of filtration in the nephron?
   a. Collecting duct → Proximal tubule → Loop of Henle
   b. Proximal tubule → Loop of Henle → Collecting duct
   c. Loop of Henle → Collecting duct → Proximal tubule
   d. Loop of Henle → Proximal tubule → Collecting duct

11. Which statement is NOT true regarding brain structure?
   a. The corpus callosum connects the hemispheres.
   b. Broca's and Wernicke's areas are associated with speech and language.
   c. The cerebellum is important for long-term memory storage.
   d. The brainstem is responsible for involuntary movement.

12. What are the functions of the hypothalamus?

   I. Regulate body temperature.
   II. Send stimulatory and inhibitory instructions to the pituitary gland.
   III. Receive sensory information from the brain.

   a. I and II
   b. I and III
   c. II and III
   d. I, II, and III

13. The somatic nervous system is responsible for which of the following?
   a. Breathing
   b. Thought
   c. Movement
   d. Fear

14. Which blood component is chiefly responsible for clotting?
   a. Platelets
   b. Red blood cells
   c. Antigens
   d. Plasma cells

15. Which is the first event to happen in a primary immune response?
   a. Macrophages ingest pathogens and present their antigens.
   b. Neutrophils aggregate and act as cytotoxic, nonspecific killers of pathogens.
   c. B lymphocytes make pathogen-specific antibodies.
   d. Helper T cells secrete interleukins to activate pathogen-fighting cells.

16. Eosinophils are best described as which of the following?
   a. A type of granulocyte that secretes histamine, which stimulates the inflammatory response
   b. The most abundant type of white blood cell, which secretes substances that are toxic to pathogens
   c. A type of granulocyte found under mucous membranes that defends against multicellular parasites
   d. A type of circulating granulocyte that is aggressive and has high phagocytic activity

17. What is an adaptation?
    a. The original traits found in a common ancestor
    b. Changes that occur in the environment
    c. When one species begins behaving like another species
    d. An inherited characteristic that enhances survival and reproduction

18. If a person with AB blood and a person with O blood have children, what is the probability that their children will have the same phenotype as either parent?
    a. 0%
    b. 25%
    c. 50%
    d. 75%

19. What does the scientific method describe?
    a. How to review a scientific paper
    b. How to organize a science laboratory
    c. The steps utilized to conduct an inquiry into a scientific question
    d. How to use science to earn money in society

20. Which element's atoms have the greatest number of electrons?
    a. Hydrogen
    b. Iron
    c. Copper
    d. Iodine

Answer Explanations #1

Reading Comprehension

1. D: This is an example of a purpose question—*why* did the author write this? The article contains facts, definitions, and other objective information without telling a story or arguing an opinion. In this case, the purpose of the article is to inform the reader. Choices *A* and *B* are incorrect because they argue for an opinion or present a position. Choice *C* is incorrect because the focus of the article is spinoff technology, not the history of space technology.

2. B: This organization question asks readers to analyze the structure of the essay. The topic of the essay is about spinoff technology, and the thesis statement at the end of the first paragraph offers the opinion, "Spinoff technology proves that it is worthwhile to invest in scientific research because it could enrich people's lives in unexpected ways." The next two paragraphs provide evidence to support this opinion, making Choice *B* the best option. Choice *A* is the second-best option because the first paragraph gives a general definition of spinoff technology, while the following two paragraphs offer more detailed examples to help illustrate this idea. However, it is not the best answer because the main idea of the essay is that spinoff technology enriches people's lives in unexpected ways. Choice *C* is incorrect because the essay does not provide details of any specific moment in history. Choice *D* is incorrect because the essay does not discuss a popular misconception.

3. C: This reading comprehension question can be answered based on the second paragraph, which describes how scientists were concerned about astronauts' nutrition and began researching useful nutritional supplements. Choice *A* in particular is not true because it reverses the order of discovery. First NASA identified the algae for astronauts to use and then it was further developed for use in baby food, not the other way around. Choices *B* and *D* are not uses of algae discussed in the article.

4. B: This vocabulary question could be answered based on the reader's prior knowledge; but even for readers who have never encountered the word "neurological" before, the passage does provide context clues. The very next sentence talks about "this algae's potential to boost brain health," which is a paraphrase of "neurological benefits." From this context, readers should be able to infer that "neurological" is related to the brain.

5. D: This question requires readers to understand the relevance of the given detail. In this case, the author mentions "costly and crucial equipment" before mentioning space suit visors, which are given as an example of something that is very valuable. Choice *A* is not correct because fashion is only related to sunglasses, not to NASA equipment. Choice *B* can be eliminated because it is simply not mentioned in the passage. While Choice *C* seems like it could be a true statement, it is also not relevant to what is being explained by the author.

6. C: The article gives several examples of how businesses have been able to capitalize on NASA research, so it is unlikely that the author would agree with this statement. Evidence for the other answer choices can be found in the article. In Choice *A,* the author mentions that "many consumers are unaware that products they are buying are based on NASA research." Choice *B* is a general definition of spinoff technology. Choice *D* is mentioned in the final paragraph.

7. D: The author mentions anti-Stratfordian arguments in the first paragraph, but then goes on to debunk these theories with more facts about Shakespeare's life in the second and third paragraphs.

Choice *A* is not correct because, while the author does present arguments from both sides, the author is far from unbiased; in fact, the author clearly disagrees with anti-Stratfordians. Choice *B* is also not correct because it is more closely aligned to the beliefs of anti-Stratfordians, whom the author disagrees with. Choice *C* can be eliminated because, while it is true that the author gives historical background, the main purpose of the article is using that information to disprove a theory.

8. B: The thesis is a statement that contains the author's topic and main idea. As seen in question 7, the main purpose of this article is to use historical evidence to provide counterarguments to anti-Stratfordians. Choice *A* is simply a definition; Choice *C* is a supporting detail, not a main idea; and Choice *D* represents an idea of anti-Stratfordians, not the author's opinion.

9. B: This question asks readers to refer to the organizational structure of the article and demonstrate understanding of how the author provides details to support their argument. This particular detail can be found in the second paragraph where the author says, "even though he did not attend university, grade-school education in Shakespeare's time was actually quite rigorous."

10. A: This is a vocabulary question that can be answered using context clues. Other sentences in the paragraph describe London as "the most populous city in England" filled with "crowds of people," giving an image of a busy city full of people. Choice *B* is not correct because London was in Shakespeare's home country, not a foreign one. Choice *C* is not mentioned in the passage. Choice *D* is not a good answer choice because the passage describes how London was a popular and important city, probably not an underdeveloped one.

11. D: Anti-Stratfordians doubt Shakespeare's ability because he was not from the upper class. His father was a glove-maker. Therefore, in at least this instance, glove-makers were not included in the upper class. This is an example of inductive reasoning, or using two specific pieces of information to draw a more general conclusion.

12. C: This detail comes from the third paragraph, where the author responds to skeptics who claim that Shakespeare wrote too much about places he never visited, so *Romeo and Juliet* is mentioned as a famous example of a play with a foreign setting. In order to answer this question, readers need to understand the author's main purpose in the third paragraph and how the author uses details to support this purpose. Choices *A* and *D* are not mentioned in the passage, and Choice *B* is not true because the passage mentions more than once that Shakespeare never left England.

13. A: This inference can be made from the final paragraph, where the author refutes anti-Stratfordian skepticism by pointing out that books about life in Europe could easily circulate throughout London. From this statement, readers can conclude that the author believes it is possible that Shakespeare learned about European culture from books, rather than visiting the continent on his own. Choice *B* is not true because the author believes that Shakespeare contributed to English literature without traveling extensively. Similarly, Choice *C* is not a good answer because the author explains how Shakespeare got his education without university. Choice *D* can also be eliminated because the author describes Shakespeare's genius, and Shakespeare was not from Italy.

14. B: "Four score and seven years ago" is the eighty-seven years, because the word "score" means "twenty."

15. D: Though the U.S. was involved in World War I and II, Choices *A* and *C* are incorrect because a civil war specifically means citizens fighting within the same country. Choice *B* is incorrect, as "the War of Spanish Succession" involved Spain, Italy, Germany, and Holland, and not the United States.

16. A: Choice *B* is incorrect because, although they are there to "dedicate a portion of that field," there is no mention in the text of an annual memorial service. Choice *C* is incorrect because there is no aggressive language in the text, only reverence for the dead. Choice *D* is incorrect because forgetting the lives that were lost is the opposite of what Lincoln is suggesting.

17. A: Choice *A* is correct because Lincoln's intention was to memorialize the soldiers who had fallen as a result of war as well as celebrate those who had put their lives in danger for the sake of their country. Choices *B* and *C* are incorrect because Lincoln's speech was supposed to foster a sense of pride among the members of the audience while connecting them to the soldiers' experiences. Choice *D* is incorrect because Lincoln is saying that the sacrifice of the soldiers is more significant than a dedication ceremony, but he doesn't suggest that the ceremony is inappropriate.

18. B: The passage begins by giving the reader information about traditional birthing situations. Then, we are told that Mr. and Mrs. Button decide to go against tradition to have their baby in a hospital. The next few paragraphs are dedicated to letting the reader know how Mr. Button dresses and goes to the hospital to welcome his new baby. There is a doctor in this excerpt, as Choice *C* indicates, and clothes are discussed, as Choice *D* indicates. However, Mr. Button is not going to the doctor's office, nor is he about to go shopping for new clothes.

19. A: We are told in the fourth paragraph that Mr. Button "arose nervously." We also see him running without caution to the doctor to find out about his wife and baby—this indicates his excitement. We also see him stuttering in a nervous yet excited fashion as he asks the doctor if it's a boy or girl. Though the doctor may seem a bit abrupt at the end, indicating a bit of anger or shame, neither of these choices is the overwhelming tone of the entire passage. Despite the circumstances, joy and gratitude are not the main tone in the passage.

20. C: The morning is *dedicated* to the birth of the Buttons' child. Choice *A, numbed*, Choice *B, chained*, and Choice *D, moved*, all could grammatically fit in the sentence. However, they do not match the excerpt's use of *consecrated* the way *dedicated* does.

21. D: The author describes a visual image—the doctor rubbing his hands together—first and foremost. The author may be trying to make a comment about the profession; however, the author does not "explain the details of the doctor's profession" as Choice *B* suggests.

22. D: We know we are being introduced to the setting because we are given the year in the very first paragraph, along with the season: "one day in the summer of 1860." This is a classic structure for an introduction of the setting. In the third paragraph we also get a long explanation of Mr. Button, who is related to him, and what his life is like.

Writing

1. A: Sentence 1 has the incorrect preposition because the word *through* is incorrectly used here. The correct preposition to describe the fact that dogs are the descendants of wolves is *from*. So, the sentence should be: While all dogs descend *from* gray wolves, it's easy to notice that dog breeds come in a variety of shapes and sizes.

2. B: The sentence should be: Selective breeding, which is also called artificial selection, is the process in which animals with desired traits are bred in order to produce offspring that share the same traits. The added commas serve to distinguish that *artificial selection* is just another term for *selective breeding* before the sentence continues. The structure is preserved, and the sentence can flow with more clarity.

3. A: Sentence 2 lacks the Oxford Comma, which helps clearly separate specific terms. The sentence should be: With such a drastic range of traits, appearances, and body types, dogs are one of the most variable and adaptable species on the planet.

4. B: *Adopt* is not the correct term. The author should have written *adapt,* because he or she is talking about how animals must modify themselves in some way to accommodate the changes in their environment. *Adopt* is to take in something as your own.

5. B: Sentence 3 has an end punctuation error because questions do not end with periods. A question mark is necessary.

6. C: Sentence 10 contains the error because the use of *into* is inappropriate for this context. The sentence should have used *on to*, describing the way genes are passed generationally.

7. D: Sentence 4 contains a subject-verb agreement error because having is singular, but the verb *are* is plural. To fix the subject-verb disagreement between the subject having *the basic knowledge* and the verb *are*, the singular is must be used in place of *are*: Rather, having the basic knowledge of how the world works, particularly how people go about gaining what they need to survive and thrive, is more important.

8. D: Sentence 1 is missing quotation marks around the quoted saying.

9. A: Sentence 1 is missing a comma after the word *goes. As the adage goes* is an introductory phrase that introduces the quote, "knowledge is power."

10. C: Sentence 11 incorrectly has the gerund, *plaguing,* instead of the past tense verb *plagued.* Recall that a gerund is a noun that is based on a verb and ends in "ing." The sentence should be: Sadly, our current society is plagued by many inconvenient truths that are attacked as lies.

11. A: Sentence 6 lacks the comma after *thinking* needed to unite the two parts of the sentence. The independent clause is *Smart leaders will engage in critical thinking*, while the dependent clause is *allowing them to discern ulterior motives and identify propaganda*. A comma is needed to effectively combine the independent clause with the dependent clause to form a complete sentence. Therefore, the sentence should be: Smart leaders will engage in critical thinking, allowing them to discern ulterior motives and identify propaganda.

12. B: Sentence 7 lacks numerical agreement between the demonstrative pronoun *these,* which is plural, and the noun *practice,* which is singular. *These* needs to be changed to *this*, making it properly modify the singular *practice*. The sentence should be: Besides catching negative intentions, this practice will serve to highlight the positives in group interactions.

13. A: Sentence 8 uses the preposition *for* instead of *to,* which is the preposition that should have been chosen. if leaders are *receptive*, they are receiving something, so *to* is appropriate.

14. B: Items in a list should be separated by a comma, and Sentence 2 is missing commas within the list to separate the items. The sentence should be: Ideally, an individual will begin their preparation for the profession in high school by taking chemistry, physics, trigonometry, and calculus.

15. B: Sentence 4 is missing an apostrophe after *one (one's).* In that sentence, the words *one* and *bachelor* need an apostrophe *-s* at the end because they show possession for the words that come after. Such curricula will aid in one's pursuit of a bachelor's degree in aircraft engineering, which requires several physical and life sciences, mathematics, and design courses.

16. C: Sentence 8 should have a comma before *which,* not a semicolon. A semicolon separates two independent clauses when a conjunction is not used, but the text that follows the semicolon here is not an independent clause. It is dependent, so a comma is needed.

17. B: Recall that prepositions are connecting words that describe relationships between other words. They are placed before a noun or pronoun, forming a phrase that modifies another word in the sentence. The preposition *of* is not required in Sentence 5. It should simply be *some universities.*

18. B: Sentence 3 is unrelated to the passage, and it interrupts the flow and continuity of the first paragraph. It needs to be deleted.

19. C: Sentence 9 has an agreement error with the demonstrative pronoun *this* and the subject *lines of work.* It should be: *Once the job begins, this line of work*. As written, *lines* does not match up with *this*; it would instead match up with the word *these*.

20. D: Sentence 12, as written, is a run-on because it connects two independent clauses with a comma without the use of a conjunction like *and* or *but* (here, *and* would have been appropriate). Otherwise, a semicolon should have been used along with a word like *additionally* to connect the two thoughts. The sentence could look something like this: As a result, aircraft engineers are compensated with generous salaries; additionally, the job outlook is good. It could also be written like this: As a result, aircraft engineers are compensated with generous salaries, and the job outlook is good.

21. A: The word *acquitted* usually means to be freed from criminal charges. The word the writer intended was *acquired* or *obtained*, or a synonym of those.

Mathematics

1. A: Converting a fraction to a percentage takes two steps. First, divide the numerator by the denominator to turn the fraction into a decimal:

$$\frac{3}{8} = 0.375$$

Now, to convert to a percentage, move the decimal point two places to the right:

$$37.5\%$$

2. A: This question involves the percent formula. Since we're beginning with a percent, also known as a number divided by 100, we'll put 39 on the right side of the equation:

$$\frac{x}{164} = \frac{39}{100}$$

Cross-multiply to get $100x = 164 \times 39 = 6{,}396$. We can solve for x by calculating $x = 6{,}396 \div 100 = 63.96$.

3. B: This question involves the percent formula.

$$\frac{32}{x} = \frac{25}{100}$$

Cross-multiply to get $25x = 32 \times 100 = 3{,}200$. We can solve for x by calculating $x = 3{,}200 \div 25 = 128$.

As an alternative, we could recall that 25% is $\frac{1}{4}$ and simply multiply 32 by 4 to get 128.

4. C: Divide 5 by 8, which results in 0.625. This rounds up to 0.63.

5. A: Divide 3 by 5 to get 0.6, and add that to the whole number, 3, to get 3.6. An alternative is to convert $3\frac{3}{5}$ to an improper fraction: $\frac{18}{5}$. Then, divide 18 by 5 to get 3.6.

6. B: $\frac{14}{25}$

Since 0.56 goes to the hundredths place, it can be placed over 100:

$$\frac{56}{100}$$

Essentially, the way to do so is by multiplying the numerator and denominator by 100:

$$\frac{0.56}{1} \times \frac{100}{100} = \frac{56}{100}$$

Then, the fraction can be simplified down to $\frac{14}{25}$:

$$\frac{56}{100} \div \frac{4}{4} = \frac{14}{25}$$

7. D: $9\frac{3}{10}$

To convert a decimal to a fraction, remember that any number to the left of the decimal point will be a whole number. Then, since 0.3 goes to the tenths place, the 3 can be placed over 10.

8. A: Using the given information of one nurse to 25 patients and 325 total patients, set up an equation to solve for number of nurses (N):

$$\frac{N}{325} = \frac{1}{25}$$

Multiply both sides by 325 to get N by itself on one side.

$$\frac{N}{1} = \frac{325}{25} = 13 \text{ nurses}$$

9. D: Using the given information of 2 beds to 1 room and 145 rooms, set up an equation to solve for the number of beds (B):

$$\frac{B}{145} = \frac{2}{1}$$

Multiply both sides by 145 to get B by itself on one side.

$$\frac{B}{1} = \frac{290}{1} = 290 \text{ beds}$$

10. C: $x = 150$

Set up the initial equation.

$$\frac{2x}{5} - 1 = 59$$

Add 1 to both sides.

$$\frac{2x}{5} - 1 + 1 = 59 + 1$$

Multiply both sides by $\frac{5}{2}$.

$$\frac{2x}{5} \times \frac{5}{2} = 60 \times \frac{5}{2} = 50$$

$$x = 150$$

11. D: Five pounds of store-brand coffee would cost $\frac{\$1.23}{1\ lbs} \times 5\ lbs = \$6.15$. Five pounds of local coffee would cost $\frac{\$1.98}{1.5\ lbs} \times 5\ lbs = \$6.60$. Calculate the price difference: $\$6.60 - \$6.15 = \$0.45$.

12. D: Find how many feet are left after the first 1,800 ft:

$$3{,}125 \text{ ft}$$

$$\underline{-1{,}800 \text{ ft}}$$

$$1{,}325 \text{ ft}$$

At $1 per foot, this part will cost $1,325. Add this to the $2,000 for the first 1,800 ft to get the total cost:

$$\$2{,}000 + \$1{,}325 = \$3{,}325$$

13. A: Figure out which is largest by looking at the first non-zero digits. Choice *B*'s first non-zero digit is in the hundredths place. The other three all have non-zero digits in the tenths place, so it must be Choice *A*, Choice *C*, or Choice *D*. Of these, Choice *A* has the largest first non-zero digit, a 4.

14. C: $40N$ would be 4,000% of N. All of the other coefficients are equivalent to $\frac{40}{100}$ or 40%.

15. A: To find the fraction of the bill that the first three people pay, the fractions need to be added, which means finding the common denominator. The common denominator is 60.

$$\frac{1}{5}+\frac{1}{4}+\frac{1}{3}=\frac{12}{60}+\frac{15}{60}+\frac{20}{60}=\frac{47}{60}$$

The remainder of the bill is:

$$1-\frac{47}{60}=\frac{60}{60}-\frac{47}{60}=\frac{13}{60}$$

16. A: The total fraction taken up by green and red shirts will be:

$$\frac{1}{3}+\frac{2}{5}=\frac{5}{15}+\frac{6}{15}=\frac{11}{15}$$

The remaining fraction is:

$$1-\frac{11}{15}=\frac{15}{15}-\frac{11}{15}=\frac{4}{15}$$

17. C: If Shawna has used $\frac{1}{3}$ of the paint, she has $\frac{2}{3}$ remaining. The mixed fraction can be converted because $2\frac{1}{2}$ gallons is the same as $\frac{5}{2}$ gallons. The calculation is:

$$\frac{2}{3}\times\frac{5}{2}=\frac{10}{6}=\frac{5}{3}=1\frac{2}{3}\text{ gallons}$$

18. D: To convert a fraction to a percent, we can first convert the fraction to a decimal. To do so, divide the numerator by the denominator: $4\div 5=0.8$. To convert a decimal to a percent, multiply by 100:

$$0.8\times 100=80\%$$

19. D: This problem can be solved using basic arithmetic. Xavier starts with 20 apples, then gives his sister half, so 20 is divided by 2.

$$\frac{20}{2}=10$$

He then gives his neighbor six apples, so 6 is subtracted from 10.

$$10-6=4$$

Finally, he uses $\frac{3}{4}$ of his remaining apples to make a pie. Since $\frac{3}{4}$ of 4 is 3, he uses 3 apples, so 3 is subtracted from 4.

$$4-3=1$$

20. B: When solving for x, add 3 to both sides to get $4x=8$. Then, divide both sides by 4 to get $x=2$.

21. A: If s is the size of the floor in square feet and r is the rate on Tuesday, then, based on the information given, $p = \frac{s}{4}$ and $r = \frac{s}{3}$. Solve the Monday rate for s, $s = 4p$, and then substitute that in the expression for Tuesday.

22. B: Using the conversion rate, multiply the projected weight loss of 25 lb by $0.45\frac{\text{kg}}{\text{lb}}$ to get the amount in kilograms (11.25 kg).

23. B: The first step is to calculate the difference between the larger value and the smaller value.

$$378 - 252 = 126$$

To calculate this difference as a percentage of the original value, and thus find the percentage increase, we calculate 126÷252=0.5. We can multiply this result by 100 to find the percentage: 50%.

24. B: Since \$850 is the price after a 20% discount, \$850 represents 80% (or 0.8) of the original price. In other words, $850 = 0.8x$ (where x is the original price). Solving this leaves the answer $x = \frac{850}{0.8} = 1{,}062.5$. Now, to find the savings, calculate the original price minus the sale price: $\$1{,}062.50 - \$850 = \$212.50$.

25. A: To determine the number of houses that can fit on the street, we can divide the length of the street by the width of each house's property:

$$345 \div 30 = 11.5$$

However, the construction company is not going to build half a house, so they will need to build either 11 or 12 houses. Since the width of 12 houses (360 feet) would extend past the length of the street, only 11 houses can be built.

26. D: A yard is 3 feet. The equation to calculate the minimum number of yards is $79 \div 3 = 26\frac{1}{3}$.

If the material is sold only by whole yards, then Mo would need to round up to the next whole yard in order to cover the extra $\frac{1}{3}$ yard. Therefore, the answer is 27 yards. None of the other choices meets the minimum whole yard requirement.

27. A: The relative error can be found by finding the absolute error and making it a percent of the true value. The absolute error is $36 - 35.75 = 0.25$. This error is then divided by 35.75—the true value—to find 0.7%.

28. A: The value went up by $\$165{,}000 - \$150{,}000 = \$15{,}000$. Out of \$150,000, this is $\frac{15{,}000}{150{,}000} = \frac{1}{10}$. If we multiply the top and bottom by 10 to give us a denominator of 100, the result is $\frac{10}{100}$, or 10%.

Science

1. D: A reflex arc is a simple nerve pathway involving a stimulus, a synapse, and a response that is controlled by the spinal cord—not the brain. The knee-jerk reflex is an example of a reflex arc. The stimulus is the hammer hitting the tendon, reaching the synapse in the spinal cord by an afferent pathway. The response is the resulting muscle contraction reaching the muscle by an efferent pathway. None of the remaining processes is a simple reflex. Memories are processed and stored in the hippocampus in the limbic system. The visual center is located in the occipital lobe, while auditory processing occurs in the temporal lobe. The sympathetic and parasympathetic divisions of the autonomic nervous system control heart rate and blood pressure.

2. A: The renal pelvis acts like a funnel by delivering the urine from the millions of collecting tubules to the ureters. It is the most central part of the kidney. The renal cortex is the outer layer of the kidney, while the renal medulla is the inner layer. The renal medulla contains the functional units of the kidneys—nephrons—which function to filter the blood. Choice *D,* Bowman's capsule, is the name for the structure that covers the glomeruli.

3. C: Capillaries are responsible for the exchange of nutrients, hormones, oxygen, fluids, and electrolytes between the blood and interstitial fluid in tissues. Hemoglobin helps carry oxygen and iron in circulating red blood cells. Arterioles and venules are intermediately sized blood vessels, but their walls are too thick for cellular-level exchange.

4. C: Although the lungs may provide some cushioning for the heart when the body is violently struck, this is not a major function of the respiratory system. Its most notable function is that of gas exchange for oxygen and carbon dioxide, but it also plays a vital role in the regulation of blood pH. The aqueous form of carbon dioxide, carbonic acid, is a major pH buffer of the blood, and the respiratory system directly controls how much carbon dioxide stays and is released from the blood through respiration. The respiratory system also enables vocalization and forms the basis for the mode of speech and language used by most humans.

5. A: The forebrain contains the cerebrum, the thalamus, the hypothalamus, and the limbic system. The limbic system is chiefly responsible for the perception of emotions through the amygdala, while the cerebrum interprets sensory input and generates movement. Specifically, the occipital lobe receives visual input, and the primary motor cortex in the frontal lobe is the controller of voluntary movement. The hindbrain, specifically the medulla oblongata and brain stem, control and regulate blood pressure and heart rate.

6. C: Nephrons are responsible for filtering blood. When functioning properly, they allow blood cells and nutrients to go back into the bloodstream while sending waste to the bladder. However, nephrons can fail at doing this, particularly when blood flow to the kidneys is limited. The medulla (also called the renal medulla) and the renal cortex are both parts of the kidney but are not specifically responsible for filtering blood. The medulla is in the inner part of the kidney and contains the nephrons. The renal cortex is the outer part of the kidney. The heart is responsible for pumping blood throughout the body rather than filtering it.

7. C: A cluster of capillaries that functions as the main filter of the blood entering the kidney is known as the glomerulus, so Choice *C* is correct. The Bowman's capsule surrounds the glomerulus and receives fluid and solutes from it; therefore, Choice *A* is incorrect. The loop of Henle is a part of the kidney tubule where water and nutrients are reabsorbed, so *B* is false. The nephron is the unit containing all of these anatomical features, making Choice *D* incorrect as well.

8. D: In the secondary immune response, suppressor T lymphocytes are activated to negate the potential risk of damage to healthy cells brought on by an unchecked, overactive immune response. Choice *A* is incorrect because this activity is characteristic of the primary response, not the secondary response. Choice *B* is incorrect because humoral immunity is mediated by antibodies produced by B, not

T, lymphocytes. Choice *C* is wrong because the secondary response is faster than the primary response because the primary response entails the time-consuming process of macrophage activation.

9. C: The parasympathetic nervous system is related to calm, peaceful times without stress that require no immediate decisions. It relaxes the fight-or-flight response, slows heart rate to a comfortable pace, and decreases bronchiole dilation to a normal size. On the other hand, the sympathetic nervous system is in charge of the fight-or-flight response and works to increase blood pressure and oxygen absorption.

10. B: Kidneys filter blood using nephrons that span the outer renal cortex and inner renal medulla. The inner kidneys are composed of the renal pelvis, which collects urine and sends it to the bladder via the ureters. Filtrate first enters the filtering tube of the nephron via the glomerulus, a bundle of capillaries where blood fluid (but not cells) diffuses into the Bowman's capsule, the entryway into the kidney filtration canal. Bowman's capsule collects fluid, but the nephron actually starts filtering blood in the proximal tubule, where necessary ions, nutrients, wastes, and (depending on blood osmolarity) water are absorbed or released. Also, blood pH is regulated here, as the proximal tubule fine-tunes pH by utilizing the blood buffering system, adjusting amounts of hydrogen ions, bicarbonate, and ammonia in the filtrate. Down the loop of Henle in the renal medulla, the filtrate becomes more concentrated as water exits. While on the way back up the loop of Henle, ion concentration is regulated with ion channels. The distal tubule continues to regulate ion and water concentrations, and the collecting duct delivers the filtrate to the renal pelvis.

11. C: The cerebellum is important for balance and motor coordination. Aside from the brainstem and cerebellum, the outside portion of the brain is the cerebrum, which is the advanced operating system of the brain that is responsible for learning, emotion, memory, perception, and voluntary movement. The amygdala (associated with emotions), language areas, and corpus callosum all exist within the cerebrum.

12. D: The hypothalamus is the link between the nervous system and the endocrine system. It receives information from the brain and sends signals to the pituitary gland, instructing it to release or inhibit the release of hormones. Aside from its endocrine function, it controls body temperature, hunger, sleep, and circadian rhythms, and it is part of the limbic system.

13. C: The somatic nervous system is the voluntary nervous system, which is responsible for voluntary movement. It includes nerves that transmit signals from the brain to the muscles of the body. Breathing is controlled by the autonomic nervous system. Thought and fear are complex processes that occur in the brain, which is part of the central nervous system.

14. A: Platelets are the blood components responsible for clotting. There are between 150,000 and 450,000 platelets in healthy blood. When a clot forms, platelets adhere to the injured area of the vessel and promote a molecular cascade that results in adherence of more platelets. Ultimately, the platelet aggregation results in recruitment of a protein called fibrin, which adds structure to the clot. Too many platelets can cause clotting disorders. Too few platelets leads to bleeding disorders.

15. A: Choice *B* might be an attractive answer choice, but neutrophils are part of the innate immune system and are not considered part of the primary immune response. The first event that happens in a primary immune response is that macrophages ingest pathogens and display their antigens. Then, they secrete interleukin 1 to recruit helper T cells. Once helper T cells are activated, they secrete interleukin 2 to stimulate plasma B and killer T cell production. Only then can plasma B make the pathogen specific antibodies.

16. C: Eosinophils, like neutrophils, basophils, and mast cells, are a type of leukocyte in a class called granulocytes. They are found underneath mucous membranes in the body and they primarily secrete destructive enzymes and defend against multicellular parasites like worms. Choice *A* describes basophils and mast cells, and Choice *B* and *D* describe neutrophils. Unlike neutrophils, which are aggressive phagocytic cells, eosinophils have low phagocytic activity.

17. D: Charles Darwin based the idea of adaptation around his original concept of natural selection. He believed that evolution occurred based on three observations: the unity of life, the diversity of life, and the suitability of organisms to their environments. There was unity in life based on the idea that all organisms descended from a common ancestor. Then, as the descendants of common ancestors faced changes in their environments or moved to new environments, they began adapting new features to help them. This concept explained the diversity of life and how organisms were matched to their environments. Natural selection helps to improve the fit between organisms and their environments by increasing the frequency of features that enhance survival and reproduction.

18. A: There is no chance that an offspring will have O blood or AB blood (see Punnett square).

	I^A	I^B
i	I^Ai	I^Bi
i	I^Ai	I^Bi

19. C: The scientific method refers to how to conduct a proper scientific inquiry, including recognizing a question/problem, formulating a hypothesis, making a prediction of what will happen based on research, experimenting, and deciding whether the outcome confirmed or denied the hypothesis.

20. D: Iodine has the greatest number of electrons at 53 electrons. The number of electrons increases in elements going from left to right across the periodic table. Hydrogen, Choice *A,* is at the top left corner of the periodic table, so it has the fewest electrons (one electron). Iron has 26 electrons, copper has 29 electrons, Choices *B* and *C*, respectively.

Practice Test #2

Reading Comprehension

Questions 1-3 are based on the following passage, which is an adaptation of Robert Louis Stevenson's The Strange Case of Dr. Jekyll and Mr. Hyde*:*

"Did you ever come across a protégé of his—one Hyde?" He asked.

"Hyde?" repeated Lanyon. "No. Never heard of him. Since my time."

That was the amount of information that the lawyer carried back with him to the great, dark bed on which he tossed to and fro until the small hours of the morning began to grow large. It was a night of little ease to his toiling mind, toiling in mere darkness and besieged by questions.

Six o'clock struck on the bells of the church that was so conveniently near to Mr. Utterson's dwelling, and still he was digging at the problem. Hitherto it had touched him on the intellectual side alone; but now his imagination also was engaged, or rather enslaved; and as he lay and tossed in the gross darkness of the night in the curtained room, Mr. Enfield's tale went by before his mind in a scroll of lighted pictures. He would be aware of the great field of lamps in a nocturnal city; then of the figure of a man walking swiftly; then of a child running from the doctor's; and then these met, and that human Juggernaut trod the child down and passed on regardless of her screams. Or else he would see a room in a rich house, where his friend lay asleep, dreaming and smiling at his dreams; and then the door of that room would be opened, the curtains of the bed plucked apart, the sleeper recalled, and, lo! There would stand by his side a figure to whom power was given, and even at that dead hour he must rise and do its bidding. The figure in these two phrases haunted the lawyer all night; and if at anytime he dozed over, it was but to see it glide more stealthily through sleeping houses, or move the more swiftly, and still the more smoothly, even to dizziness, through wider labyrinths of lamplighted city, and at every street corner crush a child and leave her screaming. And still the figure had no face by which he might know it; even in his dreams it had no face, or one that baffled him and melted before his eyes; and thus there it was that there sprung up and grew apace in the lawyer's mind a singularly strong, almost an inordinate, curiosity to behold the features of the real Mr. Hyde. If he could but once set eyes on him, he thought the mystery would lighten and perhaps roll altogether away, as was the habit of mysterious things when well examined. He might see a reason for his friend's strange preference or bondage, and even for the startling clauses of the will. And at least it would be a face worth seeing: the face of a man who was without bowels of mercy: a face which had but to show itself to raise up, in the mind of the unimpressionable Enfield, a spirit of enduring hatred.

From that time forward, Mr. Utterson began to haunt the door in the by-street of shops. In the morning before office hours, at noon when business was plenty of time scarce, at night under the face of the full city moon, by all lights and at all hours of solitude or concourse, the lawyer was to be found on his chosen post.

"If he be Mr. Hyde," he had thought, "I should be Mr. Seek."

1. What can one infer about the meaning of the word "Juggernaut" from the author's use of it in the passage?
   a. It is an apparition that appears at daybreak.
   b. It scares children.
   c. It is associated with space travel.
   d. Mr. Utterson finds it soothing.

2. What is the definition of the word *haunt* in the following passage?

> From that time forward, Mr. Utterson began to haunt the door in the by-street of shops. In the morning before office hours, at noon when business was plenty of time scarce, at night under the face of the full city moon, by all lights and at all hours of solitude or concourse, the lawyer was to be found on his chosen post.

   a. To levitate
   b. To constantly visit
   c. To terrorize
   d. To daunt

3. What can one reasonably conclude from the final comment of this passage?

> "If he be Mr. Hyde," he had thought, "I should be Mr. Seek."

   a. The speaker is considering a name change.
   b. The speaker is experiencing an identity crisis.
   c. The speaker has mistakenly been looking for the wrong person.
   d. The speaker intends to continue to look for Hyde.

Questions 4-9 are based upon the following passage:

The Myth of Head Heat Loss

It has recently been brought to my attention that most people believe that 75% of your body heat is lost through your head. I had certainly heard this before, and I'm not going to attempt to say I didn't believe it when I first heard it. It is natural to be gullible if something is said with enough authority. But the "fact" that the majority of your body heat is lost through your head is a lie.

Let me explain. Heat loss is proportional to surface area exposed. An elephant loses a great deal more heat than an anteater because it has a much greater surface area than an anteater. Each cell has mitochondria that produce energy in the form of heat, and it takes a lot more energy to run an elephant than an anteater.

So, each part of your body loses its proportional amount of heat in accordance with its surface area. The human torso probably loses the most heat, though the legs lose a significant amount as well. Some people have asked, "Why does it feel so much warmer when you cover your head than when you don't?" Well, that's because your head loses a lot of heat when it is not clothed, while the clothing on the rest of your body provides insulation. If you went outside with a hat and pants but no shirt, not only would you look stupid, but your heat loss would be significantly greater because so much more of you would be exposed. So, if given the choice to cover your chest or your head in the cold, choose the chest. It could save your life.

4. What is the primary purpose of this passage?
   a. To provide evidence that disproves a myth
   b. To compare elephants and anteaters
   c. To explain why it is appropriate to wear clothes in winter
   d. To show how people are gullible

5. Which of the following best describes the main idea of the passage?
   a. It is better to wear a shirt than a hat.
   b. Heat loss is proportional to surface area exposed.
   c. It is natural to be gullible.
   d. The human chest loses the most heat.

6. Why does the author compare elephants and anteaters?
   a. To express an opinion
   b. To give an example that helps clarify the main point
   c. To show the differences between the two
   d. To persuade why one is better than the other

7. The statement, "If you went outside with a hat and pants but no shirt, not only would you look stupid, but your heat loss would be significantly greater because so much more of you would be exposed" is which of the following?
   a. An opinion
   b. A fact
   c. An opinion within a fact
   d. Neither

8. Which of the following best describes the tone of the passage?
   a. Harsh
   b. Angry
   c. Casual
   d. Indifferent

9. Which of the following sentences provides the best evidence to support the main idea?
   a. "It is natural to be gullible if something is said with enough authority."
   b. "So, each part of your body loses its proportional amount of heat in accordance with its surface area."
   c. "So, if given the choice to cover your chest or your head in the cold, choose the chest."
   d. "But the 'fact' that the majority of your body heat is lost through your head is a lie."

Questions 10-14 are based on the following passage:

Dana Gioia argues in his article that poetry is dying, now little more than a limited art form confined to academic and college settings. Of course, poetry remains healthy in the academic setting, but the idea of poetry being limited to this academic subculture is a stretch. New technology and social networking alone have contributed to poets and other writers' work being shared across the world. YouTube has emerged to be a major asset to poets, allowing live performances to be streamed to billions of users. Even now, poetry continues to grow and voice topics that are relevant to the culture of our time. Poetry is not in the spotlight as it may have been in earlier times, but it's still a relevant art form that continues to expand in scope and appeal.

Furthermore, Gioia's argument does not account for live performances of poetry. Not everyone has taken a poetry class or enrolled in university—but most everyone is online. The Internet is a perfect launching point to get all creative work out there. An example of this was Buddy Wakefield's performance of his poem "Hurling Crowbirds at Mockingbars." Wakefield is a well-known poet who has published several collections of contemporary poetry. "Crowbirds" is one of my favorite works by Wakefield, especially because of his performance of it at New York University in 2009. Although his reading was a campus event, views of his performance online number in the thousands. His poetry attracted people outside of the university setting.

Naturally, the poem's popularity can be attributed to both Wakefield's performance and the quality of his writing. "Crowbirds" touches on themes of core human concepts such as faith, personal loss, and growth. These are not ideas that only poets or students of literature understand, but all human beings: "You acted like I was hurling crowbirds at mockingbars / and abandoned me for not making sense. / Evidently, I don't experience things as rationally as you do". Wakefield weaves together a complex description of the perplexed and hurt emotions of the speaker who is undergoing a separation from a romantic interest. The line "You acted like I was hurling crowbirds at mockingbars" conjures up an image of someone confused, seemingly out of their mind ... or in the case of the speaker, passionately trying to grasp at a relationship that is fading. The speaker is looking back and finding the words that described how he wasn't making sense. This poem is particularly human and gripping in its message, but the entire effect of the poem is enhanced through the physical performance.

At its core, poetry is about addressing issues and ideas in the world. Part of this is also addressing the perspectives that are exiguously considered. Although the platform may look different, poetry continues to have a steady audience due to the emotional connection the poet shares with the audience.

10. Which of the following best explains how the passage is organized?
    a. The author begins with a long definition of the main topic and then proceeds to prove how that definition has changed over the course of modernity.
    b. The author presents a puzzling phenomenon and uses the rest of the passage to showcase personal experiences in order to explain it.
    c. The author contrasts two different viewpoints and then builds a case showing preference for one over the other.
    d. The passage is an analysis of a theory that the author has no stake in.

11. The author of the passage would likely agree most with which of the following?
    a. Buddy Wakefield is a genius and is considered at the forefront of modern poetry.
    b. Poetry is not irrelevant; it is an art form that adapts to the changing times while retaining its core elements.
    c. Spoken word is the zenith of poetic forms and the premier style of poetry in this decade.
    d. Poetry is on the verge of vanishing from our cultural consciousness.

12. Which of the following words, if substituted for the word exiguously in the last paragraph, would LEAST change the meaning of the sentence?
    a. Indolently
    b. Inaudibly
    c. Interminably
    d. Infrequently

13. Which of the following is most closely analogous to the author's opinion of Buddy Wakefield's performance in relation to modern poetry?
    a. Someone's refusal to accept that the Higgs boson particle will validate the Standard Model of physics
    b. An individual's belief that soccer will lose popularity within the next 50 years
    c. A professor's opinion that poetry contains the language of the heart, while fiction contains the language of the mind
    d. A student's insistence that psychoanalysis is a subset of modern psychology

14. What is the primary purpose of the passage?
    a. To educate readers on the development of poetry and describe the historical implications of poetry in media
    b. To disprove Dana Gioia's stance that poetry is becoming irrelevant and is only appreciated in academia
    c. To inform readers of the brilliance of Buddy Wakefield and to introduce them to other poets that have influenced contemporary poetry
    d. To prove that Gioia's article does have some truth to it and to shed light on its relevance to modern poetry

Questions 15-18 are based upon the following passage, which is an adaptation from Mineralogy --- Encyclopedia International, Grolier

> Mineralogy is the science of minerals, which are the naturally occurring elements and compounds that make up the solid parts of the universe. Mineralogy is usually considered in terms of materials in the Earth, but meteorites provide samples of minerals from outside the Earth.

A mineral may be defined as a naturally occurring, homogeneous solid, that is inorganically formed, with a definite chemical composition, and an ordered atomic arrangement. The qualification *naturally occurring* is essential because it is possible to reproduce most minerals in the laboratory. For example, evaporating a solution of sodium chloride produces crystal indistinguishable from those of the mineral halite, but such laboratory-produced crystals are not minerals.

A *homogeneous solid* is one consisting of a single kind of material that cannot be separated into simpler compounds by any physical method. The requirement that a mineral be solid eliminates gases and liquids from consideration. Thus, ice is a mineral (a very common one, especially at high altitudes and latitudes) but water is not. Some mineralogists dispute this restriction and would consider both water and native mercury (also a liquid) as minerals.

The restriction of minerals to *inorganically formed* substances eliminates those homogenous solids produced by animals and plants. Thus, the shell of an oyster and the pearl inside, though both consist of calcium carbonate indistinguishable chemically or physically from the mineral aragonite, are not usually considered minerals.

The requirement of a *definite chemical composition* implies that a mineral is a chemical compound, and the composition of a chemical compound is readily expressed by a formula. Mineral formulas may be simple or complex, depending upon the number of elements present and the proportions in which they are combined.

Minerals are crystalline solids, and the presence of an *ordered atomic arrangement* is the criterion of the crystalline state. Under favorable conditions of formation, the ordered atomic arrangement is expressed in the external crystal form. In fact, the presence of an ordered atomic arrangement and crystalline solids was deduced from the external regularity of crystals by a French mineralogist, Abbé R. Haüy, early in the 19th century.

15. According to the text, an object or substance must have all of the following criteria to be considered a mineral EXCEPT?

a. It must be naturally occurring.
b. It must be a homogeneous solid.
c. It must be organically formed.
d. It must have a definite chemical composition.

16. One can deduce that French mineralogist Abbé R. Haüy specialized in what field of study?

a. Geology
b. Psychology
c. Biology
d. Botany

17. What is the definition of the word "homogeneous" as it appears in the following sentence?

A homogeneous solid is one consisting of a single kind of material that cannot be separated into simpler compounds by any physical method.

a. Made of a single substance
b. Differing in some areas
c. Having a higher atomic mass
d. Lacking necessary properties

18. The suffix *-logy* refers to:

a. The properties of
b. The chemical makeup of
c. The study of
d. The classification of

Questions 19-22 are based upon the following passage:

Three years ago, I think there were not many bird-lovers in the United States who believed it possible to prevent the total extinction of both egrets from our fauna. All the known rookeries accessible to plume-hunters had been totally destroyed. Two years ago, the secret discovery of several small, hidden colonies prompted William Dutcher, President of the National Association of Audubon Societies, and Mr. T. Gilbert Pearson, Secretary, to attempt the protection of those colonies. With a fund contributed for the purpose, wardens were hired and duly commissioned. As previously stated, one of those wardens was shot dead in cold blood by a plume hunter. The task of guarding swamp rookeries from the attacks of money-hungry desperadoes, to whom the accursed plumes were worth their weight in gold, is a very chancy proceeding. There is now one warden in Florida who says that "before they get my rookery they will first have to get me."

Thus far, the protective work of the Audubon Association has been successful. Now there are 20 colonies, which contain, all told, about 5,000 egrets and about 120,000 herons and ibises which are guarded by the Audubon wardens. One of the most important is on Bird Island, a mile out in Orange Lake, Central Florida, and it is ably defended by Oscar E. Baynard. To-day, the plume hunters who do not dare to raid the guarded rookeries are trying to study out the lines of flight of the birds, to and from their feeding-grounds, and shoot them in transit. Their motto is "Anything to beat the law, and get the plumes." It is there that the state of Florida should take part in the war.

The success of this campaign is attested by the fact that last year a number of egrets were seen in eastern Massachusetts—for the first time in many years. And so to-day the question is, can the wardens continue to hold the plume-hunters at bay?

Excerpt from *Our Vanishing Wild Life* by William T. Hornaday

19. What is the meaning of the word *rookeries* in the following text?

> To-day, the plume hunters who do not dare to raid the guarded rookeries are trying to study out the lines of flight of the birds, to and from their feeding-grounds, and shoot them in transit.

a. Houses in a slum area
b. A place where hunters gather to trade tools
c. A place where wardens go to trade stories
d. A colony of breeding birds

20. What is on Bird Island?
a. Hunters selling plumes
b. An important bird colony
c. Bird Island Battle between the hunters and the wardens
d. An important egret with unique plumes

21. What is the main purpose of the passage?
a. To persuade the audience to act in preservation of the bird colonies
b. To show the effect hunting egrets has had on the environment
c. To argue that the preservation of bird colonies has had a negative impact on the environment
d. To demonstrate the success of the protective work of the Audubon Association

22. Why are hunters trying to study the lines of flight of the birds?
a. To further their studies of ornithology
b. To help wardens preserve the lives of the birds
c. To have a better opportunity to hunt the birds
d. To build their homes under the lines of flight because they believe it brings good luck

Writing

Questions 1-7 are based on the following passage:

> [1]Roller skating are making a comeback as an enjoyable pastime and exercise activity. [2]Thanks to social media platforms like instagram, tiktok, and youtube, it's quicker than ever to pick up a pair of skates and learn the basics with people who are doing the same. [3]While you might see advertisements for high quality, professional skates from your favorite influencers, its easy to get intimidated by highlevel equipment. [4]If you're just starting out, you don't need a pair of skates with a high price tag. [5]A good starter pair of sturdy reliable skates can run less than \$100. [6]As you improve at skating, you'll get a better feel for your skates and learn what type of skate you might want to upgrade to. [7]You may also ask yourself, are roller skates or roller blades better? [8]Quad roller skates are traditional roller skates that feature four wheels total two on each side of the boot. [9]Quad roller skates include a brake, or toe stop, on the front toe of the boot. [10]Roller blades, or inline skates, typically feature four wheels all in a row in the center of the boot and have a brake on the heel.

1. Which sentence requires a contraction?
   a. Sentence 2
   b. Sentence 3
   c. Sentence 5
   d. Sentence 7

2. Which sentence contains a capitalization error?
   a. Sentence 2
   b. Sentence 4
   c. Sentence 6
   d. Sentence 7

3. Which sentence contains incorrect subject-verb agreement?
   a. Sentence 1
   b. Sentence 5
   c. Sentence 6
   d. Sentence 9

4. Which sentence requires a hyphen?
   a. Sentence 1
   b. Sentence 3
   c. Sentence 7
   d. Sentence 8

5. Which sentence requires a comma?
   a. Sentence 2
   b. Sentence 3
   c. Sentence 5
   d. Sentence 10

6. In which sentence is it possible to add quotation marks?
   a. Sentence 4
   b. Sentence 7
   c. Sentence 8
   d. Sentence 10

7. Which sentence is missing punctuation?
   a. Sentence 5
   b. Sentence 8
   c. Sentence 9
   d. Sentence 10

Questions 8-14 are based on the following passage:

> [1]Choosing to use roller skates or roller blades is a matter of preference because each variety of skate will provide a different expereince. [2]Quad skates are typically lighter and will provide more maneuverability. [3]Having two wheels on the front of the boot as well as two wheels on the back of the boot allows you to shift weight easily from the ball of your foot to your back heel, allowing more flexibility in turning into. [4]Roller blades,

similarly, are heavier, and the position of the wheels all in one row makes it harder to swivel on your wheels. [5]One advantage, of roller blades, is that the boot extends above the ankle and includes extra straps for security, providing for more ankle protection. [6]Some people prefer the security of roller blades and feel that they are less likely falling with the added support. [7]With the extra straps and tall boot, it is easier to feel safe. [8]Those who prefer quad skates may like neither the feel or the bulkiness of roller blades. [9]It's worth it to try both quad skates and roller blades to decide which type of skate is best for you.

8. Which sentence uses an incorrect preposition?
   a. Sentence 1
   b. Sentence 2
   c. Sentence 3
   d. Sentence 4

9. Which sentence has a spelling error?
   a. Sentence 1
   b. Sentence 2
   c. Sentence 3
   d. Sentence 4

10. Which sentence uses a comparative adverb incorrectly?
   a. Sentence 1
   b. Sentence 2
   c. Sentence 3
   d. Sentence 4

11. Which sentence uses commas incorrectly?
   a. Sentence 2
   b. Sentence 4
   c. Sentence 5
   d. Sentence 7

12. Which sentence uses an incorrect verb form?
   a. Sentence 3
   b. Sentence 6
   c. Sentence 7
   d. Sentence 9

13. Which sentence is redundant and can be eliminated from the passage?
   a. Sentence 2
   b. Sentence 4
   c. Sentence 5
   d. Sentence 7

14. Which sentence contains an error with a correlative conjunction?
    a. Sentence 3
    b. Sentence 7
    c. Sentence 8
    d. Sentence 9

Questions 15-21 are based on the following passage:

> [1]Your skates would feel well-fitted and not too tight or too loose around your feet and toes. [2]A lose skate will be difficult to balance on because your foot can slide around inside the boot while you are skating. [3] Conversely, a skate which is too tight can be painful and difficult to wear for long periods of time. [4]Both roller skates and roller blade typically include laces and sometimes have additional velcro or plastic straps to use for a tighter fit. [5]You'll want to lace their skates up as tight as you can and use the additional straps provided to minimize any looseness in your boot, while not being uncomfortable. [6]When you first try on your skates, you may want to stand on a carpet or in the grass so you can get used to balancing in them. [7]Wearing it on a non-slip surface will help you get use to the feel of your skates before you first try skating. [8]Try to shift your weight on different parts of the skate to gauge how comfortable you feel on the wheels. [9]You can even try walking around in your skates on a carpet or in the grass to get used to the extra weight on your feet. [10]Though you are probably excited to get skating, take the time to get to know your skates will help you safely transition to the pavement.

15. Which sentence uses an incorrect relative pronoun in a defining clause?
    a. Sentence 1
    b. Sentence 3
    c. Sentence 5
    d. Sentence 6

16. Which sentence contains a spelling error?
    a. Sentence 1
    b. Sentence 2
    c. Sentence 4
    d. Sentence 7

17. Which sentence contains an incorrect choice of auxiliary verb?
    a. Sentence 1
    b. Sentence 3
    c. Sentence 5
    d. Sentence 8

18. Which sentence requires a plural form of a noun?
    a. Sentence 2
    b. Sentence 3
    c. Sentence 4
    d. Sentence 5

19. Which sentence does not follow consistency in perspective?
    a. Sentence 2
    b. Sentence 5
    c. Sentence 6
    d. Sentence 8

20. Which sentence does not maintain consistency in singular vs. plural usage?
    a. Sentence 1
    b. Sentence 7
    c. Sentence 8
    d. Sentence 10

21. Which sentence contains an error in verb tense?
    a. Sentence 4
    b. Sentence 7
    c. Sentence 9
    d. Sentence 10

Mathematics

1. Which of the following numbers has the greatest value?
    a. 1.43785
    b. 1.07548
    c. 1.43592
    d. 0.89409

2. The value of 6×12 is the same as:
    a. $2 \times 4 \times 4 \times 2$
    b. $7 \times 4 \times 3$
    c. $6 \times 6 \times 3$
    d. $3 \times 3 \times 4 \times 2$

3. This chart indicates how many sales of CDs, vinyl records, and MP3 downloads occurred over the last year. Approximately what percentage of the total sales was from CDs?

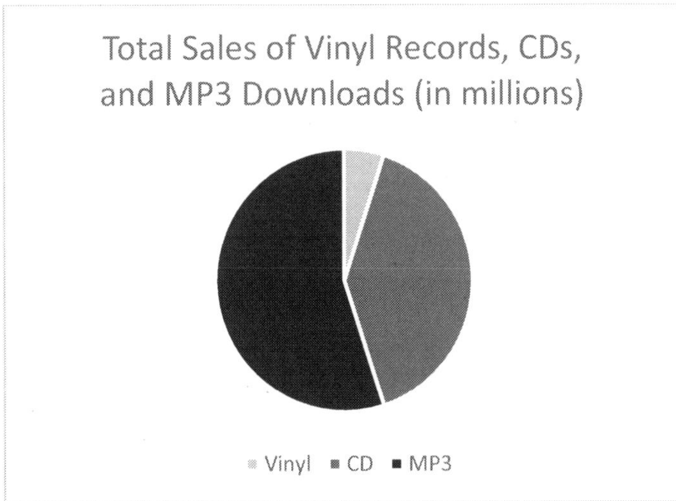

a. 55%
b. 25%
c. 40%
d. 5%

4. What is the value of b in this equation?

$$5b - 4 = 2b + 17$$

a. 13
b. 24
c. 7
d. 21

5. A school's faculty consists of 15 teachers and 20 teaching assistants. They have 200 students. What is the ratio of faculty to students?

a. $3:20$
b. $4:17$
c. $3:2$
d. $7:40$

6. Express the following in decimal form:

$$\frac{3}{5} \times \frac{7}{10} \div \frac{1}{2}$$

a. 0.042
b. 84%
c. 0.84
d. 0.42

7. A student gets an 85% on a test with 20 questions. How many questions did the student solve correctly?
   a. 15 questions
   b. 16 questions
   c. 17 questions
   d. 18 questions

8. If Sarah reads at an average rate of 21 pages in 4 nights, how long will it take her to read 140 pages?
   a. 6 nights
   b. 26 nights
   c. 8 nights
   d. 27 nights

9. Johnny earns $2,334.50 from his job each month. He pays $1,437 for monthly expenses and saves the rest. Johnny is planning a vacation in 3 months that he estimates will cost $1,750 total. How much will Johnny have left over from 3 months of saving once he pays for his vacation?
   a. $948.50
   b. $584.50
   c. $852.50
   d. $942.50

10. What is $\frac{420}{98}$ rounded to the nearest integer?
   a. 3
   b. 4
   c. 5
   d. 6

11. Give a numerical expression for the following: "Six less than three times the sum of twice a number and one."
   a. $2x + 1 - 6$
   b. $3x + 1 - 6$
   c. $3(x + 1) - 6$
   d. $3(2x + 1) - 6$

12. The total perimeter of a rectangle is 36 cm. If the length is 12 cm, what is the width?
   a. 3 cm
   b. 12 cm
   c. 6 cm
   d. 8 cm

13. Dwayne has received the following scores on his math tests: 78, 92, 83, 97. What score must Dwayne get on his next math test to have an overall average of 90?
   a. 89
   b. 98
   c. 95
   d. 100

14. What is the overall median of Dwayne's current scores: 78, 92, 83, 97?
   a. 80.5
   b. 85
   c. 90
   d. 87.5

15. Solve the following:

$$(\sqrt{36} \times \sqrt{16}) - 3^2$$

   a. 30
   b. 21
   c. 15
   d. 13

16. What is $4 \times 7 + (25 - 21)^2 \div 2$?
   a. 512
   b. 36
   c. 60.5
   d. 22

17. Kimberley earns $10 an hour babysitting, and after 10 p.m., she earns $12 an hour. The time she works is rounded to the nearest hour for pay purposes. On her last job, she worked from 5:30 p.m. to 11:00 p.m. In total, how much did Kimberley earn on her last job?
   a. $45
   b. $57
   c. $62
   d. $42

18. Solve this equation:

$$9x + x - 7 = 16 + 2x$$

   a. $x = -4$
   b. $x = 3$
   c. $x = \frac{9}{8}$
   d. $x = \frac{23}{8}$

19. Arrange the following numbers from least to greatest value: $0.85, \frac{4}{5}, \frac{2}{3}, \frac{91}{100}$
   a. $0.85, \frac{4}{5}, \frac{2}{3}, \frac{91}{100}$
   b. $\frac{4}{5}, 0.85, \frac{91}{100}, \frac{2}{3}$
   c. $\frac{2}{3}, \frac{4}{5}, 0.85, \frac{91}{100}$
   d. $0.85, \frac{91}{100}, \frac{4}{5}, \frac{2}{3}$

20. Keith's bakery had 151 customers go through its doors last week. This week, that number increased to 211. Express this increase as a percentage (round to the nearest whole number).

a. 65%
b. 40%
c. 32%
d. 76%

21. If $11x - 5 = 50$, what is the value of x?

a. 6
b. 3
c. 5
d. 4

22. Simplify the following fraction:

$$\frac{\left(\frac{5}{7}\right)}{\left(\frac{9}{11}\right)}$$

a. $\frac{55}{63}$
b. $\frac{7}{1,000}$
c. $\frac{13}{15}$
d. $\frac{5}{11}$

23. The following graph compares the various test scores of the top three students in each of these teachers' classes. Based on the graph, which teacher's students had the lowest range of test scores?

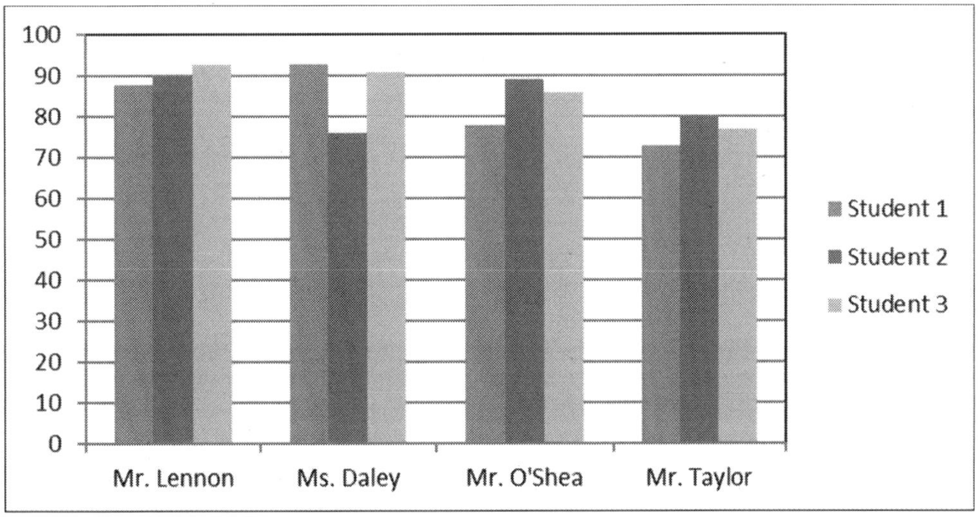

a. Mr. Lennon
b. Mr. O'Shea
c. Mr. Taylor
d. Ms. Daley

24. Bernard can make \$80 per day. If he needs to make \$300 and only works full days, how many days will this take?

a. 2 days
b. 3 days
c. 4 days
d. 5 days

25. Using the following diagram, calculate the total circumference, rounding to the nearest tenth:

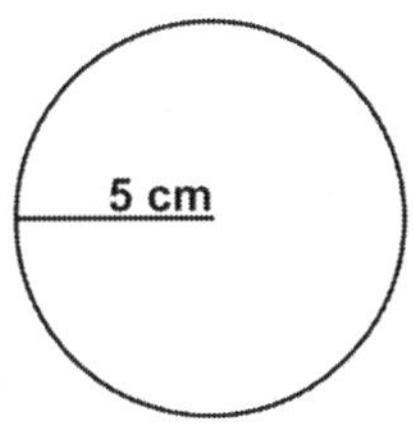

a. 25.0 cm
b. 15.7 cm
c. 78.5 cm
d. 31.4 cm

26. Which measure for the center of a small sample set would be most affected by outliers?

a. Mean
b. Median
c. Mode
d. None of the above

27. A line that travels from the lower left of a graph to the upper right of the graph indicates what kind of relationship between a predictor and a dependent variable?
   a. Positive
   b. Negative
   c. Exponential
   d. Logarithmic

28. How many kilometers is 4,382 feet if 1 foot is equal to 0.3048 meters?
   a. 1.336 kilometers
   b. 14,376 kilometers
   c. 1.437 kilometers
   d. 13,336 kilometers

Science

1. Which of the following structures is unique to eukaryotic cells?
   a. Cell walls
   b. Nuclei
   c. Cell membranes
   d. Organelles

2. Which cellular organelle is used for digestion to recycle materials?
   a. The Golgi apparatus
   b. The lysosome
   c. The centrioles
   d. The mitochondria

3. Why do arteries have valves?
   a. They have valves to maintain high blood pressure so that capillaries diffuse nutrients properly.
   b. Their valves are designed to prevent backflow due to their low blood pressure.
   c. They have valves due to a leftover trait from evolution that, like the appendix, are useless.
   d. They do not have valves, but veins do have valves.

4. If the pressure in the pulmonary artery is increased above normal, which chamber of the heart will be affected first?
   a. The right atrium
   b. The left atrium
   c. The right ventricle
   d. The left ventricle

5. Describe the synthesis of the lagging strand of DNA.
   a. DNA polymerases synthesize DNA continuously after initially attaching to a primase.
   b. DNA polymerases synthesize DNA discontinuously in pieces called Okazaki fragments after initially attaching to primases.
   c. DNA polymerases synthesize DNA discontinuously in pieces called Okazaki fragments after initially attaching to RNA primers.
   d. DNA polymerases synthesize DNA discontinuously in pieces called Okazaki fragments which are joined together in the end by a DNA helicase.

6. Using anatomical terms, what is the relationship of the sternum relative to the deltoid?
   a. Medial
   b. Lateral
   c. Superficial
   d. Posterior

7. Ligaments connect what?
   a. Muscle to muscle
   b. Bone to bone
   c. Bone to muscle
   d. Muscle to tendon

8. Identify the correct sequence of the 3 primary body planes as numbered 1, 2, and 3 in the image below.

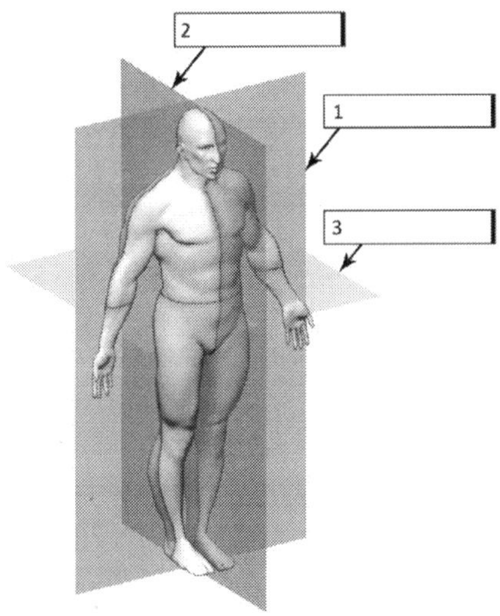

   a. Plane 1 is coronal, plane 2 is sagittal, and plane 3 is transverse.
   b. Plane 1 is sagittal, plane 2 is coronal, and plane 3 is medial.
   c. Plane 1 is coronal, plane 2 is sagittal, and plane 3 is medial.
   d. Plane 1 is sagittal, plane 2 is coronal, and plane 3 is transverse.

9. What is the major difference between somatic and germline mutations?
   a. Somatic mutations usually benefit the individual, while germline mutations usually harm them.
   b. Since germline mutations only affect one cell, they are less noticeable than the rapidly dividing somatic cells.
   c. Somatic mutations are not expressed for several generations, but germline mutations are expressed immediately.
   d. Germline mutations are usually inherited while, somatic mutations will affect only the individual.

10. A child complains of heavy breathing even when relaxing. They are an otherwise healthy child with no history of respiratory problems. What might be the issue?
   a. Asthma
   b. A blood clot
   c. Hyperventilation
   d. Exercising too hard

11. What is the purpose of a catalyst?
   a. To increase a reaction's rate by increasing the activation energy
   b. To increase a reaction's rate by increasing the temperature
   c. To increase a reaction's rate by decreasing the activation energy
   d. To increase a reaction's rate by decreasing the temperature

12. Most catalysts found in biological systems are which of the following?
   a. Special lipids called cofactors
   b. Special proteins called enzymes
   c. Special lipids called enzymes
   d. Special proteins called cofactors

13. Which of the following areas of the body has the highest density of sweat glands?
   a. Upper back
   b. Arms
   c. Palms/soles of the feet
   d. Head

14. A pediatrician notes that an infant's cartilage is disappearing and being replaced by bone. What process has the doctor observed?
   a. Mineralization
   b. Ossification
   c. Osteoporosis
   d. Calcification

15. The epidermis is composed of what type of cells?
   a. Osteoclasts
   b. Connective
   c. Dendritic
   d. Epithelial

16. Which of the following is directly transcribed from DNA and represents the first step in protein building?
   a. siRNA
   b. rRNA
   c. mRNA
   d. tRNA

17. What information does a genotype give that a phenotype does not?
    a. The genotype necessarily includes the proteins coded for by its alleles.
    b. The genotype will always show an organism's recessive alleles.
    c. The genotype must include the organism's physical characteristics.
    d. The genotype shows what an organism's parents looked like.

18. Which statement is supported by the Punnett square below, if "T" = Tall and "t" = short?

	T	*t*
T		
t		

    a. Both parents are homozygous tall.
    b. 100% of the offspring will be tall because both parents are tall.
    c. There is a 25% chance that an offspring will be short.
    d. The short allele will soon die out.

19. Which of the following is NOT found in a human cell's genes?
    a. Sequences of amino acids to be transcribed into mRNA
    b. Lethal recessive traits like sickle cell anemia
    c. Mutated DNA
    d. DNA that codes for proteins the cell doesn't use

20. Which of the following creates sperm?
    a. Prostate gland
    b. Seminal vesicles
    c. Scrotum
    d. Seminiferous tubules

Answer Explanations #2

Reading Comprehension

1. B: The passage states that the Juggernaut causes the child to scream. Choices *A* and *D* don't apply because the text doesn't mention either of these instances specifically. Choice *C* is incorrect because there is nothing in the text that mentions space travel.

2. B: The mention of *morning*, *noon*, and *night* make it clear that the word *haunt* refers to frequent appearances at various times. Choice *A* doesn't work because the text makes no mention of levitating. Choices *C* and *D* are not correct because the text makes mention of Mr. Utterson's anguish and disheartenment because of his failure to find Hyde but does not mention Mr. Utterson's feelings negatively affecting anyone else.

3. D: One can conclude that the speaker intends to continue to look for Hyde. Choices *A* and *B* are not possible answers because the text doesn't refer to any name changes or an identity crisis, despite Mr. Utterson's extreme obsession with finding Hyde. The text also makes no mention of a mistaken identity when referring to Hyde, so Choice *C* is also incorrect.

4. A: Not only does the article provide examples to disprove a myth, the title also suggests that the article is trying to disprove a myth. Further, the sentence, "But the 'fact' that the majority of your body heat is lost through your head is a lie," and then the subsequent "let me explain," demonstrates the author's intention in disproving a myth. Choice *B* is incorrect because although the selection does compare elephants and anteaters, it does so in order to prove a point, and is not the primary reason that the selection was written. Choice *C* is incorrect because even though the article mentions somebody wearing clothes in the winter, and that doing so could save your life, wearing clothes in the winter is not the primary reason this article was written. Choice *D* is incorrect because the article only mentions that people are gullible once and makes no further comment on the matter, so this cannot be the primary purpose.

5. B: If the myth is that most of one's body heat is lost through their head, then the fact that heat loss is proportional to surface area exposed is the best evidence that disproves it, since one's head is a great deal less surface area than the rest of the body, making Choice *B* the correct choice. "It is better to wear a shirt than a hat" does not provide evidence that disproves the fact that the head loses more heat than the rest of the body. Thus, Choice *A* is incorrect. Choice *C* is incorrect because gullibility is mentioned only once in this passage and the rest of the article ignores this statement, so clearly it is not the main idea. Finally, Choice *D* is incorrect because though the article mentions that the human chest probably loses the most heat, it is to provide an example of the evidence that heat loss is proportional to surface area exposed, so this is not the main idea of the passage.

6. B: Choice *B* is correct because the author is trying to demonstrate the main idea, which is that heat loss is proportional to surface area, so they compare two animals with different surface areas to clarify the main point. Choice *A* is incorrect because the author uses elephants and anteaters to prove a point that heat loss is proportional to surface area, not to express an opinion. Choice *C* is incorrect because though the author does use them to show differences, they do so in order to give examples that prove the above points. Choice *D* is incorrect because there is no language to indicate favoritism between the two animals.

7. C: Since there is an opinion presented along with a fact, Choice *C* is the correct answer. Choice *A* is incorrect. "Not only would you look stupid," is an opinion because there is no way to prove that somebody would look stupid by not wearing a shirt in the cold, even if that may be a popular opinion. However, this opinion is sandwiched inside a factual statement. Choice *B* is incorrect because again, this is a factual statement, but it has been editorialized by interjecting an opinion. Because of the presence of both a fact and an opinion, Choice *D* is the opposite of the correct answer.

8. C: Because of the way the author addresses the reader and the colloquial language the author uses (e.g., "let me explain," "so," "well," didn't," "you would look stupid," etc.), Choice *C* is the best answer because it has a much more casual tone than the usual informative article. Choice *A* may be a tempting choice because the author says the "fact" that most of one's heat is lost through their head is a "lie" and that someone who does not wear a shirt in the cold looks stupid. However, this only happens twice within the passage, and the passage does not give an overall tone of harshness. Choice *B* is incorrect because again, while not necessarily nice, the language does not carry an angry charge. The author is clearly not indifferent to the subject because of the passionate language that they use, so Choice *D* is incorrect.

9. B: The primary purpose of the article is to provide evidence to disprove the myth that most of a person's heat is lost through their head. The fact that each part of the body loses heat in proportion to its surface area is the best evidence to disprove this myth. Choice *A* is incorrect because again, gullibility is not a main contributor to this article, but it may be common to see questions on the test that give the same wrong answer in order to try and trick the test taker. Choice *C* only suggests what you should do with this information; it is not the primary evidence itself. Choice *D,* while tempting, is actually not evidence. It does not give any reason for why it is a lie; it simply states that it is. Evidence is factual information that supports a claim.

10. C: Choice *A* is incorrect because the introduction does not contain an impartial definition, but rather, an opinion. Choice *B* is incorrect. There is no puzzling phenomenon given, as the author doesn't mention any peculiar cause or effect that is in question regarding poetry. Choice *D* does contain another's viewpoint at the beginning of the passage; however, to say that the author has no stake in this argument is incorrect because the author uses personal experiences to build their case.

11. B: Choice *B* accurately describes the author's argument in the text: that poetry is not irrelevant. While the author does praise, and even value, Buddy Wakefield as a poet, the author never heralds him as a genius. Eliminate Choice *A,* as it is an exaggeration. Not only is Choice *C* an exaggerated statement, but the author never mentions spoken word poetry in the text. Choice *D* is incorrect because this statement contradicts the writer's argument.

12. D: *Exiguously* means not occurring often, or occurring rarely, so Choice *D* would least change the meaning of the sentence. Choice *A, indolently*, means unhurriedly, or slow, and does not fit the context of the sentence. Choice *B, inaudibly*, means quietly or silently. Choice *C, interminably*, means endlessly, or all the time, and is the opposite of the word *exiguously.*

13. D: A student's insistence that psychoanalysis is a subset of modern psychology is the most analogous option. The author of the passage tries to insist that performance poetry is a subset of modern poetry, and therefore, tries to prove that modern poetry is not "dying," but thriving on social media for the masses. Choice *A* is incorrect, as the author is not refusing any kind of validation. Choice *B* is incorrect; the author's insistence is that poetry will not lose popularity. Choice *C* mimics the topic but compares two different genres, making it incorrect as the author makes no comparison in this passage.

14. B: The author's purpose is to disprove Gioia's article, which claims that poetry is a dying art form that only survives in academic settings. In order to prove this argument, the author educates the reader about new developments in poetry, Choice *A*, and describes the brilliance of a specific modern poet, Choice *C*, but these serve as examples of a growing poetry trend that counters Gioia's argument. Choice *D* is incorrect because it contradicts the author's argument.

15. C: The text mentions all of the listed properties of minerals except the instance of minerals being organically formed. Objects or substances must be naturally occurring, must be a homogeneous solid, and must have a definite chemical composition in order to be considered a mineral.

16. A: Choice *A* is the correct answer because geology is the study of earth-related science. Choice *B* is incorrect because psychology is the study of the mind and behavior. Choice *C* is incorrect because biology is the study of life and living organisms. Choice *D* is incorrect because botany is the study of plants.

17. A: Choice *A* is the correct answer because the prefix *homo-* means same. Choice *B* is incorrect because "differing in some areas" would be linked to the root word *hetero-*, meaning "different" or "other."

18. C: Choice *C* is the correct answer because *-logy* refers to the study of a particular subject matter.

19. D: A *rookery* is a colony of breeding birds. Although *rookery* could mean Choice *A*, houses in a slum area, it does not make sense in this context. Choices *B* and *C* are both incorrect, as this is not a place for hunters to trade tools or for wardens to trade stories.

20. B: The previous sentence is describing "20 colonies" of birds, so what follows should be a bird colony. Choice *A* may be true, but we have no evidence of this in the text. Choice *C* does touch on the tension between the hunters and wardens, but there is no official "Bird Island Battle" mentioned in the text. Choice *D* does not exist in the text.

21. D: The text mentions several different times how and why the association has been successful and gives examples to back this fact. Choice *A* is incorrect because although the article, in some instances, calls certain people to act, it is not the purpose of the entire passage. There is no way to tell if Choices *B* and *C* are correct, as they are not mentioned in the text.

22. C: Choice *A* might be true in a general sense, but it is not relevant to the context of the text. Choice *B* is incorrect because the hunters are not studying lines of flight to help wardens, but to hunt birds. Choice *D* is incorrect because nothing in the text mentions that hunters are trying to build homes underneath lines of flight of birds for good luck.

Writing

1. B. Choice *B* is correct because Sentence 3 uses the incorrect form of the word *its*. *Its* is a possessive pronoun, whereas *it's* is a contraction for the phrase "it is." Since Sentence 3 is saying "it is easy," the contraction *it's* should be used.

2. A. Choice *A* is correct because Sentence 2 includes the proper nouns *Instagram*, *TikTok*, and *YouTube*. Since they are proper nouns that name specific social networks, they should be capitalized according to their brand names.

3. A. Choice *A* is correct because Sentence 1 starts off with the grammatically incorrect clause "Roller skating are making a comeback." Since the clause refers to the activity of roller skating, which is singular, the verb *are* must also be singular and should be corrected to *is*.

4. B. Choice *B* is correct because Sentence 3 contains the compound adjective *high-level*. Any compound adjectives that precede a noun should use a hyphen to join the adjectives.

5. C. Choice *C* is correct because Sentence 5 contains the coordinate adjectives *sturdy* and *reliable* in the phrase "sturdy reliable skates." When there is more than one adjective modifying a noun and the adjectives are of equal importance, a comma should be used to separate them. The phrase should be corrected to "sturdy, reliable adult skates."

6. B. Choice *B* is correct because Sentence 7 is posing a hypothetical question in which the reader asks themselves, "Are roller skates or roller blades better?" As a result, that clause in the sentence could be enclosed in quotation marks.

7. B. Choice *B* is correct because Sentence 8 contains the dependent clause "two on each side of the boot," which should be joined to the dependent clause with a comma or an em dash: "Quad roller skates are traditional roller skates that feature four wheels total—two on each side of the boot."

8. C. Choice *C* is correct because in Sentence 3 the preposition *into* in the phrase *turning into* should be corrected to the preposition *around*.

9. A. Choice *A* is correct because in Sentence 1, the word *experience* is spelled incorrectly.

10. D. Choice *D* is correct because Sentence 4 makes a contrast with the previous sentence, but it uses the adverb *similarly*, which instead makes a comparison and impedes the sentence's comprehensibility. The sentence can be corrected to "Roller blades, by contrast, are heavier, and the position of the wheels all in one row makes it harder to swivel on your wheels."

11. C. Choice *C* is correct because Sentence 5 incorrectly uses commas to separate out the phrase "of roller blades." Since the phrase provides context to the overarching noun phrase "One advantage of roller blades," it should not be surrounded with commas.

12. B. Choice *B* is correct because Sentence 6 uses the continuous verb form *falling* when it should use the infinitive form *to fall*. Since the verb follows the adjective phrase "less likely," the infinitive form of the verb should be used.

13. D. Choice *D* is correct because Sentence 7 states the same information as Sentence 6. As a result, it can be removed from the passage without changing what is being communicated.

14. C. Choice *C* is correct because Sentence 8 uses the correlating conjunction *neither* but follows it with the incorrect conjunction *or*. Since the conjunctions *neither* and *nor* function together as a pair, the sentence should be corrected to: "Those who prefer quad skates may like neither the feel nor the bulkiness of roller blades."

15. B. Choice *B* is correct because Sentence 3 incorrectly uses the relative pronoun *which* in the defining clause "which is too tight." Since a defining clause communicates information that is essential to the sentence, the relative pronoun *that* should be used instead: "Conversely, a skate that is too tight can be painful and difficult to wear for long periods of time."

16. B. Choice *B* is correct because Sentence 2 contains a spelling error in the word *loose*.

17. A. Choice *A* is correct because Sentence 1 uses the auxiliary verb *would*, which does not make sense in the context. *Would* is used when a sentence describes a possible situation. The auxiliary verb *should* is used when the sentence describes a recommended action, so *should* is the best auxiliary verb for this sentence: "Your skates should feel well-fitted and not too tight or too loose around your feet and toes."

18. C. Choice C is correct because Sentence 4 uses roller blade where it should use *roller blades* because of the grammatical concept of parallelism. Because *roller skates* is plural on the first side of the conjunction and, *roller blades* should match it.

19. B. Choice *B* is correct because Sentence 5 uses the second-person perspective, except for the third-person pronoun *their*. To keep the sentence consistent, *their* should be corrected to the second-person pronoun *your*.

20. B. Choice *B* is correct because Sentence 7 and the preceding sentence, Sentence 6, use the plural noun *skates*, but Sentence 7 uses the singular pronoun *it*. For consistency, Sentence 7 should use the plural pronoun *them* instead of the singular pronoun *it* when referring to the plural noun *skates*.

21. D. Choice *D* is correct because Sentence 10 uses the present tense form of the verb *take*, which makes the sentence difficult to comprehend. The sentence should use the gerund form *taking* so that it can be used as part of a noun phrase, "taking the time to get to know your skates," which goes with the verb phrase *will help*.

Mathematics

1. A: Compare each numeral after the decimal point to figure out which overall number is greatest. In Choices *A* (1.43785) and *C* (1.43592), both have the same value in the tenths (4) and hundredths (3). However, the thousandths is greater in Choice *A* (7), so *A* has the greatest value overall.

2. D: $6 \times 12 = 72$, so we can calculate the values of all four choices and find that only Choice *D* equals 72. That makes sense, because we can rearrange and group these four numbers to make the factors of the original two numbers: $(3 \times 2) \times (4 \times 3) = 6 \times 12$.

Alternatively, each of the answer choices could be prime-factored or multiplied out and compared to the original value. 6×12 has a value of 72 and a prime factorization of $2^3 \times 3^2$. The answer choices respectively have values of 64, 84, 108, and 72 and prime factorizations of 2^6, $2^2 \times 3 \times 7$, $2^2 \times 3^3$, and $2^3 \times 3^2$, so answer *D* is the correct choice.

3. C: The total percentage of a pie chart equals 100%. We can see that CD sales make up less than half of the chart (50%) but more than a quarter (25%), and the only answer choice that meets these criteria is Choice *C*, 40%.

4. C: To solve for the value of b, both sides of the equation need to be equalized. Do this by performing inverse operations to both sides of the equation.

Start by cancelling out the lower value of -4 by adding 4 to both sides:

$$5b - 4 = 2b + 17$$

$$5b - 4 + 4 = 2b + 17 + 4$$

$$5b = 2b + 21$$

The variable b is the same on each side, so subtract the lower $2b$ from each side:

$$5b = 2b + 21$$

$$5b - 2b = 2b + 21 - 2b$$

$$3b = 21$$

Then divide both sides by 3 to get the value of b:

$$3b = 21$$

$$\frac{3b}{3} = \frac{21}{3}$$

$$b = 7$$

5. D: The total faculty is $15 + 20 = 35$. So, the ratio is $35 : 200$. Then, divide both of these numbers by 5, since 5 is a common factor to both, with a result of $7 : 40$.

6. C: The first step in solving this problem is expressing the result in fraction form. We can start by performing the division operation on the last two fractions. When dividing one fraction by another, invert—or flip—the second fraction and then multiply the numerators and denominators.

$$\frac{7}{10} \times \frac{2}{1} = \frac{14}{10}$$

Next, multiply the first fraction by this value:

$$\frac{3}{5} \times \frac{14}{10} = \frac{42}{50}$$

In this instance, to find the decimal form, we can multiply the numerator and denominator by 2 to get 100 in the denominator.

$$\frac{42}{50} \times \frac{2}{2} = \frac{84}{100}$$

In decimal form, this would be expressed as 0.84.

7. C: To find what 85% of 20 questions is, multiply 20 by 0.85:

$$20 \text{ x } .85 = 17 \text{ questions}$$

8. D: This problem can be solved by setting up a proportion involving the given information and the unknown value. The proportion is:

$$\frac{21 \text{ pages}}{4 \text{ nights}} = \frac{140 \text{ pages}}{x \text{ nights}}$$

Cross-multiply to get $21x = 4 \times 140$. Solving this leaves $x \approx 26.67$. Since this is not an integer, round up to 27 nights because 26 nights would not give Sarah enough time to finish.

9. D: First, subtract $1,437 from $2,334.50 to find Johnny's monthly savings; this equals $897.50. Then, multiply this amount by 3 to find out how much he will have (in 3 months) before he pays for his vacation; this equals $2,692.50. Finally, subtract the cost of the vacation ($1,750) from this amount to find how much Johnny will have left: $942.50.

10. B: Dividing by 98 can be approximated by dividing by 100, which would mean shifting the decimal point of the numerator to the left by 2. The result is 4.2, which rounds to 4.

11. D: "Sum" means the result of addition, so "the sum of twice a number and one" can be written as 2x+1. Next, "three times the sum of twice a number and one" would be $3(2x + 1)$. Finally, "six less than three times the sum of twice a number and one" would be $3(2x + 1) - 6$.

12. C: The formula for the perimeter of a rectangle is $P = 2l + 2w$, where P is the perimeter, l is the length, and w is the width. The first step is to substitute all of the data into the formula:

$$36 = 2(12) + 2w$$

Simplify by multiplying 2×12:

$$36 = 24 + 2w$$

Simplifying this further by subtracting 24 on each side, which gives:

$$36 - 24 = 24 - 24 + 2w$$

$$12 = 2w$$

Divide by 2:

$$6 = w$$

The width is 6 cm. Remember to test this answer by substituting this value into the original formula:

$$36 = 2(12) + 2(6)$$

13. D: To find the average of a set of values, add the values together and then divide by the total number of values. In this case, include the unknown value, x, of what Dwayne needs to score on his next test. The average must equal 90. Set up the equation and solve:

First, combine like terms:

$$\frac{78 + 92 + 83 + 97 + x}{5} = 90$$

$$\frac{350 + x}{5} = 90$$

Next, multiply both sides by 5:

$$(5)\frac{350 + x}{5} = (90)(5)$$

$$350 + x = 450$$

Lastly, subtract 350 from both sides:

$$350 + x - 350 = 450 - 350$$

$$x = 100$$

14. D: For an even number of total values, the *median* is calculated by finding the *mean* or average of the two middle values once all values have been arranged in order from least to greatest. In this case, $\frac{83+92}{2}$ would equal the median 87.5, Choice *D*.

15. C: Follow the *order of operations* in order to solve this problem. Solve the parentheses first, and then follow the remainder as usual.

$$(6 \times 4) - 9$$

This equals 24 − 9 or 15, answer *C*.

16. B: To solve this correctly, keep in mind the order of operations with the mnemonic PEMDAS (Please Excuse My Dear Aunt Sally). This stands for Parentheses, Exponents, Multiplication & Division, Addition & Subtraction. Taking it step by step, start with the parentheses:

$$4 \times 7 + (4)^2 \div 2$$

Then, apply the exponent:

$$4 \times 7 + 16 \div 2$$

Multiplication and division are both performed next:

$$28 + 8 = 36$$

17. C: Kimberley worked 4.5 hours at the rate of $\frac{\$10}{\text{h}}$ and 1 hour at the rate of $\frac{\$12}{\text{h}}$. The problem states that her time is rounded to the nearest hour, so the 4.5 hours would round up to 5 hours at the rate of $\frac{\$10}{\text{h}}$.

$$(5\text{ hours}) \times \left(\frac{\$10}{\text{hour}}\right) + (1\text{ hour}) \times \left(\frac{\$12}{\text{hour}}\right) = \$50 + \$12 = \$62$$

18. D:

$9x + x - 7 = 16 + 2x$	Combine $9x$ and x.
$10x - 7 = 16 + 2x$	
$10x - 7 + 7 = 16 + 2x + 7$	Add 7 to both sides to remove the −7.
$10x = 23 + 2x$	
$10x - 2x = 23 + 2x - 2x$	Subtract $2x$ from both sides to move it to the other side of the equation.
$8x = 23$	
$\frac{8x}{8} = \frac{23}{8}$	Divide by 8 to get x by itself.
$x = \frac{23}{8}$	

19. C: For each fraction, we can divide the numerator by the denominator to find a decimal value. $4/5 = 0.8, \frac{2}{3} \approx 0.67, and \frac{91}{100} = 0.91$. Ordering these from least to greatest gives us 0.67, 0.8, 0.85, and 0.91, which matches Choice *C*.

20. B: First, calculate the difference between the larger value and the smaller value:

$$211 - 151 = 60$$

To calculate this difference as a percentage of the original value, which is the percentage *increase*, divide 60 by 151 to get 0.3974, then multiply by 100 to reach the percentage 39.74%. Rounding to the nearest whole number makes the answer 40%, Choice *B*.

21. C: To solve for x in $11x - 5 = 50$, the variable must be isolated. Start by adding 5 to both sides.

$$11x - 5 + 5 = 50 + 5$$

$$11x = 55$$

Then divide both sides by 11.

$$\frac{11}{11}x = \frac{55}{11} = 5$$

The answer is $x = 5$.

22. A: First, simplify the larger fractions by separating it into two. When dividing one fraction by another, remember to invert the second fraction and multiply the two as follows:

$$\frac{5}{7} \div \frac{9}{11} = \frac{5}{7} \times \frac{11}{9}$$

The resulting fraction $\frac{55}{63}$ cannot be simplified further, so this is the answer to the problem.

23. A: To calculate the range in a set of data, subtract the lowest value from the highest value. In this graph, the range of Mr. Lennon's students is 4, which can be seen physically in the graph as having the smallest difference between the highest value and the lowest value compared with the other teachers.

24. C: The number of days can be found by taking the total amount Bernard needs to make and dividing it by the amount he earns per day:

$$\frac{300}{80} = \frac{30}{8} = \frac{15}{4} = 3.75$$

Bernard will need to work four days since he is only working full days and three days is not enough time.

25. D: To calculate the circumference of a circle, use the formula $2\pi r$, where r equals the radius or half of the diameter of the circle and $\pi = \sim 3.14$. Substitute the given information, $2\pi 5 = 31.4$, answer *D*.

26. A: An outlier is a data value that's either far above or below the majority of values in a sample set. The mean is the average of all values in the set. In a small sample, a very high or low number could greatly change the average. The median is the middle value when arranged from lowest to highest. Outliers would have no more of an effect on the median than any other value. Mode is the value that repeats most often in a set. Assuming that the same outlier doesn't repeat, outliers would have no effect on the mode of a sample set.

27. A: This vector indicates a positive relationship. A negative relationship would show points traveling from the top-left of the graph to the bottom-right. Exponential and logarithmic functions aren't linear (don't create a straight line), so these options could have been immediately eliminated.

28. A: The conversion can be obtained by setting up and evaluating the following expression:

$$4{,}382 \text{ ft} \times \frac{0.3048 \text{ m}}{1 \text{ ft}} \times \frac{1 \text{ km}}{1{,}000 \text{ m}} = 1.336 \text{ km}$$

Science

1. B: The structure exclusively found in eukaryotic cells is the nucleus. Animal, plant, fungi, and protist cells are all eukaryotic. DNA is contained within the nucleus of eukaryotic cells, and they also have membrane-bound organelles that perform complex intracellular metabolic activities. Prokaryotic cells (archaea and bacteria) do not have a nucleus or other membrane-bound organelles and are less complex than eukaryotic cells.

2. B: The cell structure responsible for cellular storage, digestion, and waste removal is the lysosome. Lysosomes are like recycle bins. They are filled with digestive enzymes that facilitate catabolic reactions to regenerate monomers. The Golgi apparatus is designed to tag, package, and ship out proteins destined for other cells or locations. The centrioles typically play a large role only in cell division when they ratchet the chromosomes from the mitotic plate to the poles of the cell. The mitochondria are involved in energy production and are the powerhouses of the cell.

3. D: Veins have valves, but arteries do not. Valves in veins are designed to prevent backflow since they are the furthest blood vessels from the pumping action of the heart and steadily increase in volume (which decreases the available pressure). Capillaries diffuse nutrients properly because of their thin walls and high surface area and are not particularly dependent on positive pressure.

4. C: The blood leaves the right ventricle through a semi-lunar valve and goes through the pulmonary artery to the lungs. Any increase in pressure in the artery will eventually affect the contractibility of the right ventricle. Blood enters the right atrium from the superior and inferior venae cavea veins, and blood leaves the right atrium through the tricuspid valve to the right ventricle. Blood enters the left atrium from the pulmonary veins carrying oxygenated blood from the lungs. Blood flows from the left atrium to the left ventricle through the mitral valve and leaves the left ventricle through a semi-lunar valve to enter the aorta.

5. C: The lagging strand of DNA falls behind the leading strand because of its discontinuous synthesis. DNA helicase unzips the DNA helices so that synthesis can take place, and RNA primers are created by the RNA primase for the polymerases to attach to and build from. The lagging strand is synthesizing DNA in a direction that is hard for the polymerase to build, so multiple primers are laid down so that the entire length of DNA can be synthesized simultaneously. These short pieces of DNA being synthesized are known as Okazaki fragments and are joined together by DNA ligase.

6. A: The sternum is medial to the deltoid because it is much closer (typically right on) the midline of the body, while the deltoid is lateral at the shoulder cap. Superficial means that a structure is closer to the body surface and posterior means that it falls behind something else. For example, skin is superficial to bone and the kidneys are posterior to the rectus abdominis.

7. B: Ligaments connect bone to bone. Tendons connect muscle to bone. Both are made of dense, fibrous connective tissue (primarily type I collagen) to give strength. However, tendons are more organized, especially in the long axis direction like muscle fibers themselves, and they have more collagen. This arrangement makes sense because muscles have specific orientations of their fibers, so they contract in somewhat predictable directions. Ligaments are less organized and have more of a woven pattern because bone connections are not as organized as bundles or muscle fibers, so ligaments must have strength in multiple directions to protect against injury.

8. A: The three primary body planes are coronal, sagittal, and transverse. The coronal or frontal plane, named for the plane in which a corona or halo might appear in old paintings, divides the body vertically into front and back sections. The sagittal plane, named for the path an arrow might take when shot at the body, divides the body vertically into right and left sections. The transverse plane divides the body horizontally into upper or superior and lower or inferior sections. There is no medial plane, per se. The anatomical direction medial simply references a location close or closer to the center of the body than another location.

9. D: Germline mutations in eggs and sperm are permanent, can be on the chromosomal level, and will be inherited by offspring. Somatic mutations cannot affect eggs and sperm, and therefore are not inherited by offspring. Mutations of either kind are rarely beneficial to the individual but do not necessarily harm them. Germline cells divide much more rapidly than do somatic cells, and a mutation in a sex cell would promulgate and affect many thousands of its daughter cells.

10. A: It is most likely asthma. Any of the answer choices listed can cause heavy breathing. A blood clot in the lung (*B*) could cause this, but this would be very uncommon for a child. Choices *C* and *D* can both be ruled out because the question mentions that it occurs even when the patient is relaxing. Hyperventilation is usually caused by a panic attack or some sort of physical activity. Asthma often develops during childhood. It would stand to reason then that the child may have not yet been diagnosed. While asthma attacks can be caused by exercise, they can also occur when a person is not exerting themselves.

11. C: A catalyst functions to increase reaction rates by decreasing the activation energy required for a reaction to take place. Inhibitors would increase the activation energy or otherwise stop the reactants from reacting. Although increasing the temperature usually increases a reaction's rate, this is not true in all cases, and most catalysts do not function in this manner.

12. B: Biological catalysts are termed *enzymes*, which are proteins with conformations that specifically manipulate reactants into positions which decrease the reaction's activation energy. Lipids do not usually affect reactions, and cofactors, while they can aid or be necessary to the proper functioning of enzymes, do not make up the majority of biological catalysts.

13. C: The relative density of eccrine sweat glands varies in different areas of the body. The palms and soles of the feet have the highest density, reaching values of approximately 400 sweat glands per square centimeter of epidermis. The head also has a high density of sweat glands, though significantly less than on the palms and soles. Areas such as the upper arms and thighs have only around 80 eccrine sweat glands per square inch of skin.

14. B: Ossification is the process by which cartilage, a soft, flexible substance is replaced by bone throughout the body. All humans regardless of age have cartilage, but cartilage in some areas is replaced by bones as a person grows.

15. D: The outermost layer of the skin, the epidermis, consists of epithelial cells. This layer of skin is dead, as it has no blood vessels. Osteoclasts are cells that make up bones. Notice the prefix "osteo-," which means bone. Connective tissue macrophage cells can be found in a variety of places, and dendritic cells are part of the lymphatic system.

16. C: mRNA is directly transcribed from DNA before being taken to the cytoplasm and translated by rRNA into a protein. tRNA transfers amino acids from the cytoplasm to the rRNA for use in building these proteins. siRNA is a special type of RNA which interferes with other strands of mRNA, typically by causing them to get degraded by the cell rather than translated into protein.

17. B: Since the genotype is a depiction of the specific alleles that an organism's genes code for, it includes recessive genes that may or may not be otherwise expressed. The genotype does not have to name the proteins that its alleles code for; indeed, some of them may be unknown. The phenotype is the physical, visual manifestations of a gene, not the genotype. The genotype does not necessarily include any information about the organism's physical characteristics. Although some information about an organism's parents can be obtained from its genotype, its genotype does not actually show the parents' phenotypes.

18. C: One in four offspring (or 25%) will be short, so all four offspring cannot be tall. Although both of the parents are tall, they are hybrid or heterozygous tall, not homozygous. A Punnett square cannot determine if a short allele will die out. Although it may seem intuitive that the short allele will be expressed by lower numbers of the population than the tall allele, it still appears in 75% of the offspring (although its effects are masked in $\frac{2}{3}$ of those). Besides, conditions could favor the recessive allele and kill off the tall offspring.

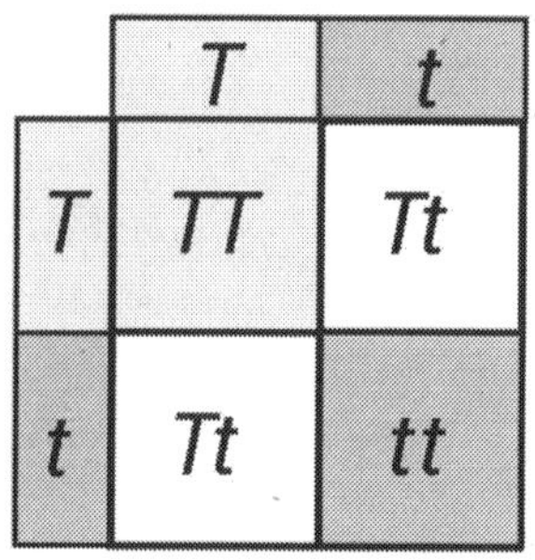

Both parents are mixed hybrids so offspring are a 3:1 ratio

19. A: Human genes are strictly DNA and do not include proteins or amino acids. A human's genome and collection of genes will include even their recessive traits, mutations, and unused DNA.

20. D: The seminiferous tubules are responsible for sperm production. Had *testicles* been an answer choice, it would also have been correct since it houses the seminiferous tubules. The prostate gland (*A*) secretes enzymes that help nourish sperm after creation. The seminal vesicles (*B*) secrete some of the components of semen. The scrotum (*C*) is the pouch holding the testicles.

Practice Test #3

Reading Comprehension

Questions 1-4 are based on the following passage:

> Smoking tobacco products is terribly destructive. A single cigarette contains over 4,000 chemicals, including 43 known carcinogens and 400 deadly toxins. Some of the most dangerous ingredients include tar, carbon monoxide, formaldehyde, ammonia, arsenic, and DDT. Smoking can cause numerous types of cancer, including throat, mouth, nasal cavity, esophageal, gastric, pancreatic, renal, bladder, and cervical cancer.
>
> Cigarettes contain a drug called nicotine, one of the most addictive substances known. Addiction is defined as a compulsion to seek the substance despite negative consequences. According to the National Institute on Drug Abuse, nearly 35 million smokers expressed a desire to quit smoking in 2015; however, more than 85% of those who struggle with addiction will not achieve their goal. Almost all smokers regret picking up that first cigarette. You would be wise to learn from their mistake if you have not yet started smoking.
>
> According to the US Department of Health and Human Services, 16 million people in the United States presently suffer from a smoking-related condition, and nearly nine million suffer from a serious smoking-related illness. According to the Centers for Disease Control and Prevention (CDC), tobacco products cause nearly six million deaths per year. This number is projected to rise to over eight million deaths by 2030. Smokers, on average, die ten years earlier than their nonsmoking peers.
>
> In the United States, local, state, and federal governments typically tax tobacco products, which leads to high prices. Nicotine users who struggle with addiction sometimes pay more for a pack of cigarettes than for a few gallons of gas. Additionally, smokers tend to stink. The smell of smoke is all-consuming and creates a pervasive nastiness. Smokers also risk staining their teeth and fingers with yellow residue from the tar.
>
> Smoking is deadly, expensive, and socially unappealing. Clearly, smoking is not worth the risks.

1. Which of the following best describes the passage?
    a. Narrative
    b. Persuasive
    c. Expository
    d. Technical

2. Which of the following statements most accurately summarizes the passage?
    a. Tobacco is less healthy than many alternatives.
    b. Tobacco is deadly, expensive, and socially unappealing, and smokers would be much better off kicking the addiction.
    c. In the United States, local, state, and federal governments typically tax tobacco products, which leads to high prices.
    d. Tobacco products shorten smokers' lives by ten years and kill more than six million people per year.

3. The author would be most likely to agree with which of the following statements?
    a. Smokers should only quit cold turkey and should avoid all nicotine cessation devices.
    b. Other substances are more addictive than tobacco.
    c. Smokers should quit for whatever reason gets them to stop smoking.
    d. People who want to continue smoking should advocate for a reduction in tobacco product taxes.

4. Which of the following represents an opinion statement on the part of the author?
    a. According to the Centers for Disease Control and Prevention (CDC), tobacco products cause nearly six million deaths per year.
    b. Nicotine patches are just as terrible as cigarettes.
    c. Smokers also risk staining their teeth and fingers with yellow residue from the tar.
    d. Additionally, smokers tend to stink. The smell of smoke is all-consuming and creates a pervasive nastiness.

Questions 5-7 are based on the following passage:

George Washington emerged out of the American Revolution as an unlikely champion of liberty. On June 14, 1775, the Second Continental Congress created the Continental Army, and John Adams, serving in the Congress, nominated Washington to be its first commander. Washington had fought under the British during the French and Indian War, and his experience and prestige proved instrumental to the American war effort. Washington provided invaluable leadership, training, and strategy during the Revolutionary War. He emerged from the war as the embodiment of liberty and freedom from tyranny.

After vanquishing the heavily favored British forces, Washington could have pronounced himself the autocratic leader of the former colonies without any opposition, but he famously refused and returned to his Mount Vernon plantation. His restraint proved his commitment to the fledgling state's republicanism. Washington was later unanimously elected as the first American president. But it is Washington's farewell address that cemented his legacy as a visionary worthy of study.

In 1796, President Washington issued his farewell address by public letter. Washington enlisted his good friend, Alexander Hamilton, in drafting his most famous address. The letter expressed Washington's faith in the Constitution and rule of law. He encouraged his fellow Americans to put aside partisan differences and establish a national union. Washington warned Americans against meddling in foreign affairs and entering military alliances. Additionally, he stated his opposition to national political parties, which he considered partisan and counterproductive.

Americans would be wise to remember Washington's farewell, especially during presidential elections, when politics hit a fever pitch. They might want to question the political institutions that were not planned by the Founding Fathers, such as the nomination process and political parties themselves.

5. Which of the following statements is logically based on the information contained in the passage above?
   a. George Washington's background as a wealthy landholder directly led to his faith in equality, liberty, and democracy.
   b. George Washington would have opposed America's involvement in the Second World War.
   c. George Washington would not have been able to write as great a farewell address without the assistance of Alexander Hamilton.
   d. George Washington would probably not approve of modern political parties.

6. Which of the following is the best description of the author's purpose in writing this passage about George Washington?
   a. To inform American voters about a Founding Father's sage advice on a contemporary issue and explain its applicability to modern times
   b. To introduce George Washington to readers as a historical figure worthy of study
   c. To note that George Washington was more than a famous military hero
   d. To convince readers that George Washington is a hero of republicanism and liberty

7. In which of the following materials would the author be the most likely to include this passage?
   a. A history textbook
   b. An obituary
   c. A fictional story
   d. A newspaper editorial

Questions 8-10 are based upon the following passage:

This excerpt is adapted from "The 'Hatchery' of the Sun-Fish"— Scientific American, #711

I have thought that an example of the intelligence (instinct?) of a class of fish which has come under my observation during my excursions into the Adirondack region of New York State might possibly be of interest to your readers, especially as I am not aware that anyone except myself has noticed it, or, at least, has given it publicity.

The female sun-fish (called, I believe, in England, the roach or bream) makes a "hatchery" for her eggs in this wise. Selecting a spot near the banks of the numerous lakes in which this region abounds, and where the water is about 4 inches deep, and still, she builds, with her tail and snout, a circular embankment 3 inches in height and 2 thick. The circle, which is as perfect a one as could be formed with mathematical instruments, is usually a foot and a half in diameter; and at one side of this circular wall an opening is left by the fish of just sufficient width to admit her body.

The mother sun-fish, having now built or provided her "hatchery," deposits her spawn within the circular enclosure, and mounts guard at the entrance until the fry are hatched out and are sufficiently large to take charge of themselves. As the embankment, moreover, is built up to the surface of the water, no enemy can very easily obtain an entrance within the enclosure from the top; while there being only one entrance, the fish is able, with comparative ease, to keep out all intruders.

I have, as I say, noticed this beautiful instinct of the sun-fish for the perpetuity of her species more particularly in the lakes of this region; but doubtless the same habit is common to these fish in other waters.

8. What is the purpose of this passage?
   a. To show the effects of fish hatcheries on the Adirondack region
   b. To persuade the audience to study ichthyology (fish science)
   c. To depict the sequence of mating among sun-fish
   d. To enlighten the audience on the habits of sun-fish and their hatcheries

9. What does the word *wise* in this passage most closely mean?
   a. Knowledge
   b. Manner
   c. Shrewd
   d. Ignorance

10. What is the definition of the word *fry* as it appears in the following passage?

    The mother sun-fish, having now built or provided her "hatchery," deposits her spawn within the circular enclosure, and mounts guard at the entrance until the fry are hatched out and are sufficiently large to take charge of themselves.

   a. Fish at the stage of development where they are capable of feeding themselves
   b. Fish eggs that have been fertilized
   c. A place where larvae are kept out of danger from other predators
   d. A dish where fish are placed in oil and fried until golden brown

Questions 11-17 are based upon the following passage:

The Global Water Crisis

For decades, the world's water supply has been decreasing. At least 10% of the world's population, or over 780 million people, does not have access to potable water. They have to walk for miles, carrying heavy buckets in intense heat, in order to obtain the essential life source that comes freely from our faucets.

We are in a global water crisis. Only 2.5% of the water on Earth is suitable for drinking, and over 70% of this water is frozen in the polar ice caps or located deep underground. This leaves a very small percentage available for drinking, yet we see millions of gallons of water wasted on watering huge lawns in deserts like Arizona, or on running dishwashers that are only half-full, or on filling all the personal pools in Los Angeles; meanwhile, people in Africa are dying of thirst.

In order to reduce water waste, Americans and citizens of other industrialized countries should adhere to the following guidelines: run the dishwasher only when it is full, do only full loads of laundry, wash the car with a bucket and not with a hose, take showers only when necessary, swim in public pools, and just be cognizant of how much water they are using in general. Our planet is getting thirstier by the year, and if we do not solve this problem, our species will surely perish.

11. Which of the following best supports the assertion that we need to limit our water usage?
    a. People are wasting water on superfluous things.
    b. There is very little water on Earth suitable for drinking.
    c. At least 10% of the world population does not have access to drinking water.
    d. There is plenty of drinking water in industrialized countries but not anywhere else.

12. How is the content in the selection organized?
    a. In chronological order
    b. Compare and contrast
    c. As a set of problems and solutions
    d. As a series of descriptions

13. Which of the following, if true, would challenge the assertion that we are in a global water crisis?
    a. There are abundant water stores on Earth that scientists are not reporting.
    b. Much of the water we drink comes from rain.
    c. People in Africa only have to walk less than a mile to get water.
    d. Most Americans only run the dishwasher when it is full.

14. The selection is written in which of the following styles?
    a. As a narrative
    b. In a persuasive manner
    c. As an informative piece
    d. As a series of descriptions

15. Which of the following is implicitly stated within the following sentences?

    This leaves a very small percentage available for drinking, yet we see millions of gallons of water wasted on watering huge lawns in deserts like Arizona, or on running dishwashers that are only half-full, or on filling all the personal pools in Los Angeles; meanwhile people in Africa are dying of thirst.

    a. People run dishwashers that are not full.
    b. People in Africa are dying of thirst.
    c. People take water for granted.
    d. People should stop watering their lawns.

16. Why does the author mention that people have to walk for miles in intense heat to get water?
    a. To inform the reader on the hardships of living with water scarcity
    b. To inspire compassion in the reader
    c. To show that water is only available in industrialized countries
    d. To persuade the reader to reduce their water usage

17. What is the main idea of the passage?
    a. People should reduce their water usage.
    b. There is very little drinking water on earth.
    c. People take their access to water for granted.
    d. People should swim in public pools.

Questions 18–22 are based upon the following passage:

> My gentleness and good behaviour had gained so far on the emperor and his court, and indeed upon the army and people in general, that I began to conceive hopes of getting my liberty in a short time. I took all possible methods to cultivate this favourable disposition. The natives came, by degrees, to be less apprehensive of any danger from me. I, Gulliver, would sometimes lie down, and let five or six of them dance on my hand; and at last, the boys and girls would venture to come and play at hide-and-seek in my hair. I had now made a good progress in understanding and speaking the language. The emperor had a mind one day to entertain me with several of the country shows, wherein they exceed all nations I have known, both for dexterity and magnificence. I was diverted with none so much as that of the rope-dancers, performed upon a slender white thread, extended about two feet, and twelve inches from the ground. Upon which I shall desire liberty, with the reader's patience, to enlarge a little.
>
> This diversion is only practised by those persons who are candidates for great employments, and high favour at court. They are trained in this art from their youth, and are not always of noble birth, or liberal education. When a great office is vacant, either by death or disgrace (which often happens), five or six of those candidates petition the emperor to entertain his majesty and the court with a dance on the rope; and whoever jumps the highest, without falling, succeeds in the office. Very often the chief ministers themselves are commanded to show their skill, and to convince the emperor that they have not lost their faculty. Flimnap, the treasurer, is allowed to cut a caper on the straight rope, at least an inch higher than any other lord in the whole empire. I have seen him do the summerset several times together, upon a trencher fixed on a rope which is no thicker than a common packthread in England. My friend Reldresal, principal secretary for private affairs, is, in my opinion, if I am not partial, the second after the treasurer; the rest of the great officers are much upon a par.
>
> Excerpt adapted from Gulliver's Travels into Several Remote Nations of the World by Jonathan Swift

18. Which of the following statements best summarizes the central purpose of this text?
    a. Gulliver details his fondness for the archaic, yet interesting, practices of his captors.
    b. Gulliver conjectures about the intentions of the aristocratic sector of society.
    c. Gulliver becomes acquainted with the people and practices of his new surroundings.
    d. Gulliver's differences cause him to become penitent around new acquaintances.

19. What is the word *principal* referring to in the following text?

> My friend Reldresal, principal secretary for private affairs, is, in my opinion, if I am not partial, the second after the treasurer; the rest of the great officers are much upon a par.

a. Primary or chief
b. An acolyte
c. An individual who provides nurturing
d. One in a subordinate position

20. What can the reader infer from this passage?

> I, Gulliver, would sometimes lie down, and let five or six of them dance on my hand; and at last, the boys and girls would venture to come and play at hide-and-seek in my hair.

a. Gulliver traveled because he wanted to meet new people.
b. The children tortured Gulliver.
c. Gulliver is considerably larger than the children who are playing around him.
d. Gulliver has a genuine love and enthusiasm for people of all sizes.

21. What is the significance of the word *mind* in the following passage?

> The emperor had a mind one day to entertain me with several of the country shows, wherein they exceed all nations I have known, both for dexterity and magnificence.

a. The ability to think
b. A collective vote
c. A definitive decision
d. A mythological question

22. Which of the following assertions does not support the fact that games are a commonplace event in this culture?

a. My gentleness and good behavior ... short time.
b. They are trained in this art from their youth ... liberal education.
c. Very often the chief ministers themselves are commanded to show their skill ... not lost their faculty.
d. Flimnap, the treasurer, is allowed to cut a caper on the straight rope ... higher than any other lord in the whole empire.

Writing

Questions 1-7 are based on the following passage:

> [1]A powerful but solitary creature, the Snow Leopard is one of the last big cats of Asia. [2]Making its habitat across twelve countrys, the snow leopard resides in rocky, high-altitude mountain regions, mostly along the Himalayan mountain range in China and Nepal and extending into the Middle East. [3]However, the snow leopard was known to make its home as far north as Mongolia and southern Russia. [4]These animals live alone for their adult lives and are most active hunting in the early morning or late evening. [5]Despite living on steep outcrops the snow leopard is quite nimble and can cover a large distance in a short amount of time. [6]Scientists have reported that

female snow leopards can require as much as fifty square miles of habitat, with male snow leopards requiring as many as one hundred square miles. [7]Snow leopards will mark there territory with urine or pheromones, warning others to stay away and only coming together to mate. [8]Female snow leopards will typically give birth to a litter of two to three cubs and raise the cubs for one to two years. [9]In captivity, the oldest snow leopard lived to be twenty-one years old, but in the wild, the snow leopards lifespan is considered to be half as long due to harsh survival conditions and threat of poaching.

1. Which sentence has a spelling error and requires a possessive pronoun?
   a. Sentence 3
   b. Sentence 5
   c. Sentence 6
   d. Sentence 7

2. Which sentence has an error with verb tense?
   a. Sentence 1
   b. Sentence 3
   c. Sentence 5
   d. Sentence 6

3. Which sentence has a capitalization error?
   a. Sentence 1
   b. Sentence 2
   c. Sentence 4
   d. Sentence 6

4. Which sentence has an incorrect spelling of a plural noun?
   a. Sentence 1
   b. Sentence 2
   c. Sentence 3
   d. Sentence 5

5. Which sentence has a punctuation error?
   a. Sentence 3
   b. Sentence 4
   c. Sentence 5
   d. Sentence 8

6. Which sentence has an error with an adjective that describes a plural noun?
   a. Sentence 2
   b. Sentence 6
   c. Sentence 7
   d. Sentence 9

7. Which sentence has an error with possession?
   a. Sentence 1
   b. Sentence 4
   c. Sentence 6
   d. Sentence 9

Questions 8-14 are based on the following passage:

> [1]Measuring up to five feet long and weighing up to 120 pounds, the snow leopard is distinctive for its smoke-colored coat and black spots. [2]The mottled fur helps it camouflage against the snow and rock of its mountain habitat. [3]The coat is also incredibly thin and protects the snow leopard from frigid temperatures reaching as low as negative forty degrees Fahrenheit. [4]The snow leopard has a tail that is nearly as long as its body and giant, padded paws. [5]Its tail helps it keep its balance when jumping along the mountainous cliffs, and its paws help to muffle its movements when it is stalking prey. [6]For food, the snow leopard feasts on a variety of mountain-dwelling sheep and goats. [7]Such as bharal and mountain ibex, as well as small mammals and birds. [8]Like many big, carnivorous cats, it is at the mercy of the hunt and could go days without having a meal. [9]When it finally catches its prey, it will eat its fill and conserve its energy by lounging or to nap in a secluded spot until it needs to venture out again.

8. Which sentence has an adjective that makes the sentence difficult to comprehend?
   a. Sentence 1
   b. Sentence 2
   c. Sentence 3
   d. Sentence 4

9. Which sentence requires a correction to its punctuation?
   a. Sentence 3
   b. Sentence 4
   c. Sentence 6
   d. Sentence 8

10. Which sentence is a fragment that should be combined with an earlier sentence?
    a. Sentence 5
    b. Sentence 7
    c. Sentence 8
    d. Sentence 9

11. Where should the following sentence be inserted to make the most sense and aid the flow of the paragraph?

    > Snow leopards are impressive predators and can kill prey that weigh up to three times their body weight.

    a. After Sentence 1
    b. After Sentence 3
    c. After Sentence 4
    d. After Sentence 5

12. Which sentence requires a hyphen?
    a. Sentence 1
    b. Sentence 3
    c. Sentence 4
    d. Sentence 8

13. Which sentence uses the incorrect verb tense?
    a. Sentence 5
    b. Sentence 6
    c. Sentence 8
    d. Sentence 9

14. Which sentence contains an error in verb consistency?
    a. Sentence 3
    b. Sentence 4
    c. Sentence 6
    d. Sentence 9

Questions 15-21 are based on the following passage:

> [1]The snow leopard has long been victim to poaching, illegal capture and trade as an exotic pet, and destroying of its habitat by climate change and by humans for livestock production. [2]As a result, it has been placed it under a protective status of "vulnerable" by the international union for conservation of nature, or IUCN. [3]As of the year twenty twenty-two, there are thought to be less than 7,000 snow leopards worldwide and its population continues to decrease under time. [4]The snow leopard is legally classified as protected animal in many Asian countries and there are punishments like imprisonment and fines for illegal hunting and trading it. [5]In 2013, the Global Snow Leopard Forum was formed and government leaders made a comitmment to work together to boost protection efforts for the snow leopard. [6]The use of non-invasive methods to study wild snow leopards is costly however scientists are committed to it. [7]Zoos also continue fund breeding research and programs in hopes of restoring the population.

15. Which sentence contains a spelling error?
    a. Sentence 2
    b. Sentence 3
    c. Sentence 4
    d. Sentence 5

16. Which sentence uses a gerund incorrectly?
    a. Sentence 1
    b. Sentence 2
    c. Sentence 5
    d. Sentence 6

17. Which sentence should use a numeral?
    a. Sentence 1
    b. Sentence 3
    c. Sentence 4
    d. Sentence 7

18. Which sentence has a capitalization error?
    a. Sentence 1
    b. Sentence 2
    c. Sentence 3
    d. Sentence 4

19. Which sentence uses an adjective that should instead be an adverb?
   a. Sentence 4
   b. Sentence 5
   c. Sentence 6
   d. Sentence 7

20. Which sentence requires an infinitive?
   a. Sentence 2
   b. Sentence 3
   c. Sentence 5
   d. Sentence 7

21. Which sentence is a run-on sentence that needs correct punctuation?
   a. Sentence 1
   b. Sentence 3
   c. Sentence 4
   d. Sentence 6

Mathematics

1. Which of the following is the best description of the relationship between x and y?

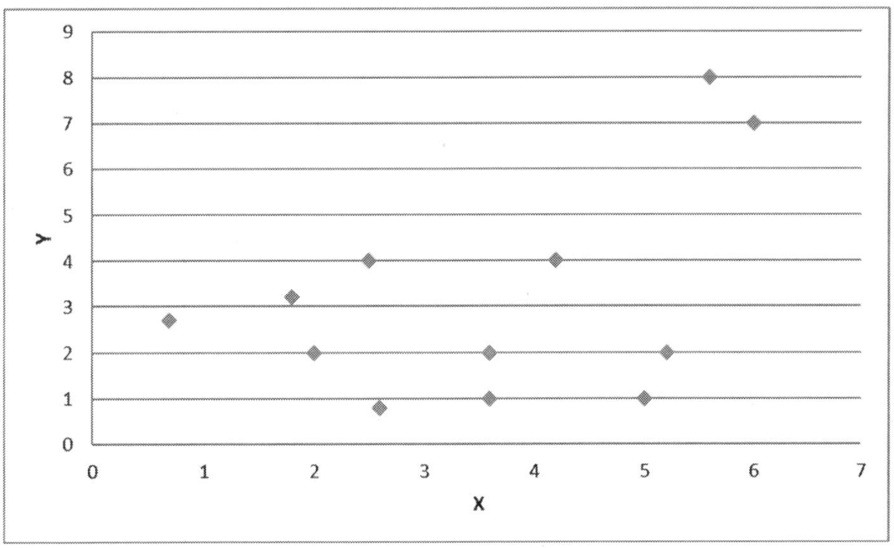

   a. The data has normal distribution.
   b. x and y have a negative relationship.
   c. x and y have no apparent relation.
   d. x and y have a positive relationship.

2. What is the slope of this line?

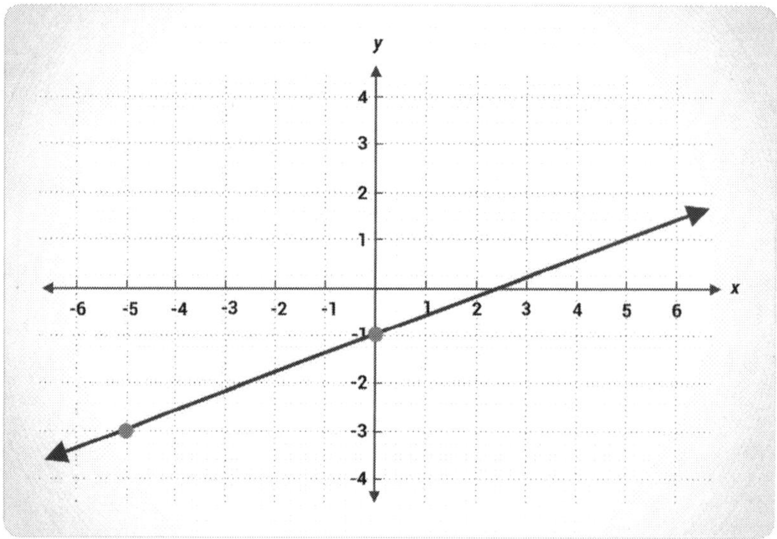

a. 2

b. $\frac{5}{2}$

c. $\frac{1}{2}$

d. $\frac{2}{5}$

3. What is the perimeter of the figure below? Note that the solid outer line is the perimeter.

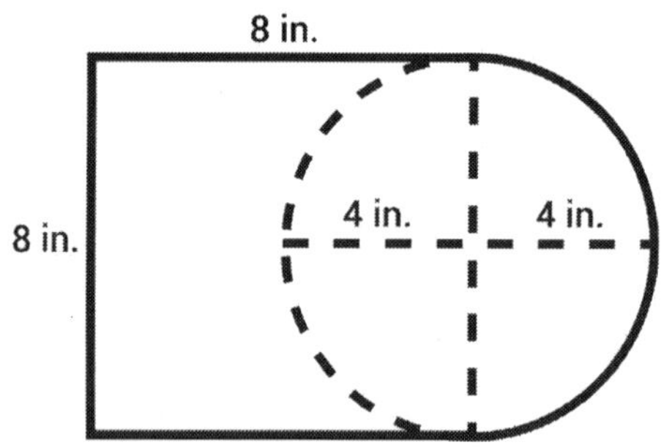

a. 48.565 in
b. 36.565 in
c. 39.78 in
d. 39.565 in

4. Which of the following equations best represents the problem below?

> The width of a rectangle is 2 centimeters less than the length. If the perimeter of the rectangle is 44 centimeters, then what are the dimensions of the rectangle?

a. $2l + 2(l - 2) = 44$
b. $(l + 2) + (l + 2) + l = 48$
c. $l \times (l - 2) = 44$
d. $(l + 2) + (l + 2) + l = 44$

5. Which of the following is the result of simplifying the expression: $\frac{4a^{-1}b^3}{a^4b^{-2}} \times \frac{3a}{b}$?

a. $12a^3b^5$
b. $12\frac{b^4}{a^4}$
c. $\frac{12}{a^4}$
d. $7\frac{b^4}{a}$

6. What is the product of two irrational numbers?

a. Irrational
b. Rational
c. Irrational or rational
d. Complex and imaginary

7. The graph shows the position of a car over a 10-second time interval. Which of the following is the correct interpretation of the graph for the interval 1 to 3 seconds?

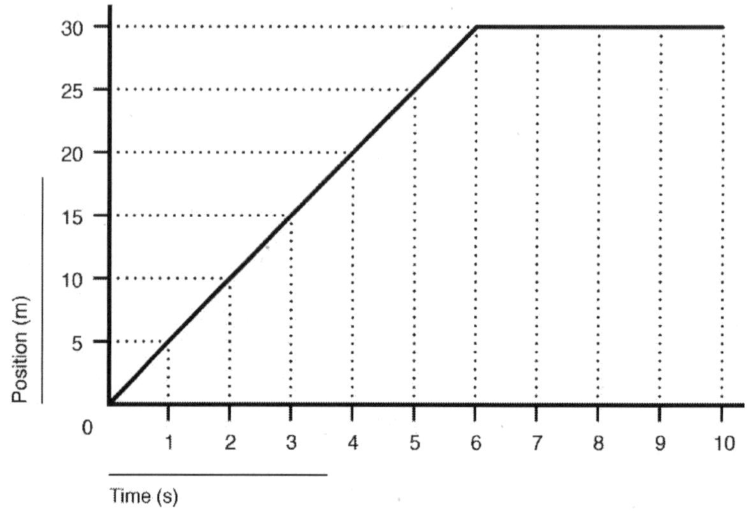

a. The car remains in the same position.
b. The car is traveling at a speed of 5 m/s.
c. The car is traveling up a hill.
d. The car is traveling at 5 mph.

8. The number –4 can be classified as which of the following?
a. Real, rational, integer, whole, natural
b. Real, rational, integer, natural
c. Real, rational, integer
d. Real, irrational

9. $4\frac{1}{3} + 3\frac{3}{4} =$

a. $6\frac{5}{12}$

b. $8\frac{1}{12}$

c. $8\frac{2}{3}$

d. $7\frac{7}{12}$

10. Five of six numbers have a sum of 25. The average of all six numbers is 6. What is the sixth number?
a. 8
b. 10
c. 11
d. 12

11. 4.67 miles is equivalent to how many kilometers, to three significant digits? Use the conversion $1\ \text{mi} = 1.609\ \text{km}$.

a. 7.514 km
b. 7.51 km
c. 2.90 km
d. 2.902 km

12. If $\frac{5}{2} \div \frac{1}{3} = n$, then n is between:

a. 5 and 7
b. 7 and 9
c. 9 and 11
d. 3 and 5

13. What are all the factors of 12?

a. 12, 24, 36
b. 1, 2, 4, 6, 12
c. 12, 24, 36, 48
d. 1, 2, 3, 4, 6, 12

14. How would the number 847.89632 be written if rounded to the nearest hundredth?

a. 847.90
b. 900
c. 847.89
d. 847.896

15. What is the value of the sum of $\frac{1}{3}$ and $\frac{2}{5}$?

a. $\frac{3}{8}$
b. $\frac{11}{15}$
c. $\frac{11}{30}$
d. $\frac{4}{5}$

16. Add and express in reduced form: $\frac{5}{12} + \frac{4}{9}$

a. $\frac{9}{17}$
b. $\frac{1}{3}$
c. $\frac{31}{36}$
d. $\frac{3}{5}$

17. Divide and reduce: $\frac{4}{13} \div \frac{27}{169}$
   a. $\frac{52}{27}$
   b. $\frac{51}{27}$
   c. $\frac{52}{29}$
   d. $\frac{51}{29}$

18. Express the following as a reduced mixed number: $\frac{54}{15}$.
   a. $3\frac{3}{5}$
   b. $3\frac{1}{15}$
   c. $3\frac{3}{54}$
   d. $3\frac{1}{54}$

19. In the problem $5 \times 6 + 4 \div 2 - 1$, which operation should be completed first?
   a. Multiplication
   b. Addition
   c. Division
   d. Subtraction

20. Express the following as an improper fraction: $8\frac{3}{7}$.
   a. $\frac{11}{7}$
   b. $\frac{21}{8}$
   c. $\frac{5}{3}$
   d. $\frac{59}{7}$

21. Express the following as an improper fraction: $11\frac{5}{8}$.
   a. $\frac{55}{8}$
   b. $\frac{93}{8}$
   c. $\frac{16}{11}$
   d. $\frac{19}{5}$

22. Round to the nearest tenth: 8.067.
   a. 8.07
   b. 8.1
   c. 8.00
   d. 8.11

23. When rounding 245.2678 to the nearest thousandth, which place value would be used to decide whether to round up or round down?
   a. Ten-thousandths
   b. Thousandths
   c. Hundredths
   d. Thousands

24. Simplify $(1.2 \times 10^{12} \div 3.0 \times 10^{8})$ and write the result in scientific notation.
   a. 0.4×10^4
   b. 4.0×10^4
   c. 4.0×10^3
   d. 3.6×10^{20}

25. The phone bill is calculated each month using the equation $c = 50g + 75$. The cost of the phone bill per month is represented by c, and g represents the gigabytes of data used that month. What is the value and interpretation of the slope of this equation?
   a. 75 dollars per day
   b. 75 gigabytes per day
   c. 50 dollars per day
   d. 50 dollars per gigabyte

26. Mom's car drove 72 miles in 90 minutes. How fast did she drive in feet per second?
   a. 0.8 feet per second
   b. 48.9 feet per second
   c. 0.009 feet per second
   d. 70.4 feet per second

27. $3\frac{2}{3} - 1\frac{4}{5} =$
   a. $1\frac{13}{15}$
   b. $\frac{14}{15}$
   c. $2\frac{2}{3}$
   d. $\frac{4}{5}$

28. 20 is 40% of what number?
   a. 50
   b. 8
   c. 200
   d. 5,000

Science

1. What is the sensory threshold?
   a. The smallest amount of stimulus required for an individual to feel a sensation
   b. The amount of stimulus required for an individual to feel pain
   c. The amount of stimulus required to cause an individual to move away from the stimulus
   d. The place where the stimulus is coming from

2. How many neurons generally make up a sensory pathway?
   a. 1
   b. 2
   c. 3
   d. 4

3. In which part of the eye does visual processing begin?
   a. Cornea
   b. Optic nerve
   c. Retina
   d. Eyelid

4. What type of vessel carries oxygen-rich blood from the heart to other tissues of the body?
   a. Veins
   b. Intestines
   c. Bronchioles
   d. Arteries

5. The process of breaking down large molecules into smaller molecules to provide energy is known as which of the following?
   a. Metabolism
   b. Bioenergetics
   c. Anabolism
   d. Catabolism

6. Which of the following correctly lists the four properties that all types of muscle tissue share?
   a. Contractile, excitable, elastic, extensible
   b. Contractile, voluntary, elastic, extensible
   c. Contractile, excitable, voluntary, extensible
   d. Contractile, excitable, elastic, voluntary

7. Which of the following statements about the autonomic nervous system (ANS) is true?
   a. It controls the reflex arc.
   b. It contains motor (efferent) neurons.
   c. It contains sensory (afferent) neurons.
   d. It contains both parasympathetic nerves and sympathetic nerves.

8. What is the function of the sinuses?
   a. To trap the many airborne pathogens
   b. To direct air down the trachea rather than the esophagus
   c. To warm, humidify, and filter air
   d. To sweep away pathogens and direct them toward the top of the trachea

9. Which of the following is the body cavity that contains the urinary bladder, urethra, and ureters?
   a. The thoracic cavity
   b. The pelvic cavity
   c. The abdominal cavity
   d. The spinal cavity

10. What is an alteration in the normal gene sequence called?
   a. DNA mutation
   b. Gene migration
   c. Polygenetic inheritance
   d. Incomplete dominance

11. Blood type is a trait determined by multiple alleles, and two of them are co-dominant: I^A codes for A blood and I^B codes for B blood. The i allele codes for O blood and is recessive to both. If an A heterozygous individual and an O individual have a child, what is the probability that the child will have A blood?
   a. 25%
   b. 50%
   c. 75%
   d. 100%

12. With which genotype would the recessive phenotype appear, if the dominant allele is marked with A and the recessive allele is marked with a?
   a. AA
   b. aa
   c. Aa
   d. aA

13. What is the name for the structural and functional units located in the cortex of the kidney that create and transport urine?
   a. Glomerulus
   b. Nephrons
   c. Loops of Henle
   d. Distal tubules

14. The muscular tube that connects the outer surface to the cervix in a woman's birth canal is referred to as which of the following?
   a. The uterus
   b. The cervix
   c. The vagina
   d. The ovaries

15. Which of the following hormones is primarily responsible for regulating metabolism?
    a. Insulin
    b. Testosterone
    c. Adrenaline
    d. Thyroid hormone

16. Which of the following is the gland that helps regulate calcium levels?
    a. Osteoid gland
    b. Pineal gland
    c. Parathyroid glands
    d. Thymus gland

17. What makes bone resistant to shattering?
    a. The calcium salts deposited in the bone
    b. The collagen fibers
    c. The bone marrow and network of blood vessels
    d. The intricate balance of minerals and collagen fibers

18. What is the name for the sac-shaped structures that facilitate the exchanging of carbon dioxide and oxygen?
    a. Kidneys
    b. Medulla oblongata
    c. Alveoli
    d. Bronchioles

19. Which of the following organs functions as both an endocrine and exocrine gland?
    a. The kidney
    b. The spleen
    c. The pancreas
    d. The stomach

20. Which of the following systems does NOT include a transportation system throughout the body?
    a. Cardiovascular system
    b. Endocrine system
    c. Immune system
    d. Nervous system

Answer Explanations #3

Reading Comprehension

1. B: Narrative, Choice *A,* means a written account of connected events. Think of narrative writing as a story. Choice C, expository writing, generally seeks to explain or describe some phenomenon, whereas Choice D, technical writing, includes directions, instructions, and/or explanations. This passage is persuasive writing, which hopes to change someone's beliefs based on an appeal to reason or emotion. The author is aiming to convince the reader that smoking is terrible. They use health, price, and beauty in their argument against smoking, so Choice *B,* persuasive, is the correct answer.

2. B: The author cites disease and deaths associated with smoking, and points to the monetary expense and aesthetic costs. Choice *A* is wrong because alternatives to smoking are not addressed in the passage. Choice *C* is wrong because it does not summarize the passage but rather is just a premise. Choice *D* is wrong because, while these statistics are a premise in the argument, they do not represent a summary of the piece. Choice *B* is the correct answer because it states the three critiques offered against tobacco and expresses the author's conclusion.

3. C: We are looking for something the author would agree with, so it should be anti-smoking or an argument in favor of quitting smoking. Choice *A* is wrong because the author does not speak against means of cessation. Choice *B* is wrong because the author does not reference other substances but does speak of how addictive nicotine, a drug in tobacco, is. Choice *D* is wrong because the author would not encourage reducing taxes to encourage a reduction of smoking costs, thereby helping smokers to continue the habit. Choice *C* is correct because the author is attempting to persuade smokers to quit smoking.

4. D: Here, we are looking for the author's opinion rather than a fact or statistic. Choice *A* is wrong because quoting statistics from the CDC is stating facts, not opinions. Choice *B* is wrong because it expresses the fact that cigarettes sometimes cost more than a few gallons of gas. It would be an opinion if the author said that cigarettes were not affordable. Choice *C* is incorrect because yellow stains are a known possible adverse effect of smoking. Choice *D* is correct as an opinion because smell is subjective. Some people might like the smell of smoke, they might not have working olfactory senses, and/or some people might not find the smell of smoke akin to "pervasive nastiness," so this is the expression of an opinion. Thus, Choice *D* is the correct answer.

5. D: Although Washington was from a wealthy background, the passage does not say that his wealth led to his republican ideals, so Choice *A* is not supported. Choice *B* also does not follow from the passage. Washington's warning against meddling in foreign affairs does not mean that he would oppose wars of every kind, so Choice *B* is wrong. Choice *C* is also unjustified since the author does not indicate that Alexander Hamilton's assistance was absolutely necessary. Choice *D* is correct because the passage states that Washington's farewell address clearly opposes political parties and partisanship. The author then notes that presidential elections often hit a fever pitch of partisanship. Thus, it follows that George Washington would probably not approve of modern political parties and their involvement in presidential elections.

6. A: The author finishes the passage by applying Washington's farewell address to modern politics, so the purpose probably includes this application. The other descriptions also fit the passage to some degree, but they do not describe the author's main purpose, which is revealed in the final paragraph.

7. D: Choice *A* is wrong because the last paragraph is not appropriate for a history textbook. Choice *B* is false because the piece is not a notice or announcement of Washington's death. Choice *C* is false because it is not fiction, but a historical writing. Choice *D* is correct. The passage is most likely to appear in a newspaper editorial because it cites information that is relevant and applicable to the present day, a popular subject in editorials.

8. D: *A* is incorrect because although the Adirondack region is mentioned in the text, there are no cause or effect relationships between the region and fish hatcheries depicted here. Choice *B* is incorrect because the text does not have an agenda, but rather is meant to inform the audience. Finally, Choice *C* is incorrect because the text says nothing of how sun-fish mate.

9. B: The word *wise* in this passage most closely means *manner*. Choices *A* and *C* are synonyms of *wise*; however, they are not relevant in the context of the text. Choice *D, ignorance*, is opposite of the word wise and is therefore incorrect.

10. A: Even if the word *fry* isn't immediately known to the reader, the context gives a hint when it says "until the fry are hatched out and are sufficiently large to take charge of themselves."

11. B: Choice *B* is correct because having very little drinking water on Earth is a very good reason that one should limit their water usage so that the human population does not run out of drinking water and die out. People wasting water on superfluous things does not support the argument that we need to limit our water usage. It merely states that people are wasteful. Therefore, Choice *A* is incorrect. Answer Choice *C* may be tempting, but it is not the correct one, as this article is not about reducing water usage in order to help those who don't have easy access to water. It is about the fact that the planet is running out of drinking water. Choice *D* is incorrect because nowhere in the article does it state that only industrialized countries have access to drinking water.

12. C: The primary purpose is to present a problem (the planet is running out of water) with a solution (reduce water waste); therefore, the correct answer is Choice *C*. Choice *A* is incorrect because the passage does not have a sequential timeline of events and is therefore not in chronological order. It may be tempting to think the author compares and contrasts people who do not have access to drinking water to those who do, but that does not fit with the primary purpose of the article, which is to convince people to reduce their water usage. Thus, Choice *B* is incorrect. Choice *D* is incorrect because descriptions are not the primary content of this article. Remember that a descriptive writing style describes people, settings, or situations in great detail with many adjectives. While a descriptive writing voice may be used alongside a persuasive writing style, it is generally not the primary voice when trying to convince a reader to take a certain stance.

13. A: If the assertion is that the Earth does not have enough drinking water, then having abundant water stores that are not being reported would certainly challenge this assertion. Choice *B* is incorrect because even if much of the water we drink does come from rain, that means the human population would be dependent on rain in order to survive, which would support the assertion instead of challenge it. the primary purpose of the passage is not to help those who cannot get water, then Choice *C* is not the correct answer. Even if Choice *D* were true, it does not dismiss the other ways in which people are wasteful with water, and it is also not the point.

14. B: Choice *B* is correct because the article uses a lot of emotionally charged language and also suggests what needs to be done with the information provided. The article does not contain elements of a narrative, which include plot, setting, characters, and themes. Not only does the article lack these things, but it does not follow a timeline, which is a key element of a narrative voice. Thus, Choice *A* is incorrect. Choice *C* is incorrect because the article uses information in order to be persuasive, but the purpose is not solely to inform on the issue. Choice *D* is incorrect because the article is not written in primarily descriptive language.

15. C: Choice *C* is correct because people who waste water on lawns in the desert, or run a half-full dishwasher, or fill their personal pools are not taking into account how much water they are using because they get an unlimited supply; therefore, they are taking it for granted. Choices *A* and *B* are incorrect because they are both explicitly stated within the given sentences. As for Choice *D*, the passage may imply that people should water their lawns less, but not necessarily that they need to stop altogether.

16. B: Choice *B* is correct because the author uses this example in order to show people, through emotional appeal, that they take water for granted because they get water freely from their faucets, while millions of people have to endure great hardships to get drinking water. Choice *A* does not pertain directly to the main idea of the article, nor does it pertain to the author's purpose. The main idea is that people should reduce their water usage, and the author's purpose is to persuade the reader to do so. Choice *C* is incorrect because the selection never mentions that water is only available in industrialized countries. Choice *D* is the author's purpose for the entire passage but not the purpose for mentioning the difficulty in getting water for some of the population.

17. A: Choice *B* is a reason that people should reduce their water usage, but it is not the main idea. Choice *C* is an explanation for water waste but, again, not the main idea. Choice *D* is a suggestion for reducing water usage but still not the main idea.

18. C: Choice *C* is the correct answer because it most extensively summarizes the entire passage. While Choices *A* and *B* are reasonable possibilities, they reference portions of Gulliver's experience, not the whole. Choice *D* is incorrect because Gulliver doesn't express repentance or sorrow in this particular passage.

19. A: Principal refers to *chief* or *primary* within the context of this text. Choice *A* is the answer that most closely aligns with this definition. Choices *B* and *D* refer to a helper or follower, while Choice *C* doesn't meet the description of Reldresal from the passage.

20. C: One can reasonably infer that Gulliver is considerably larger than the children who were playing around him because multiple children could fit into his hand. Choice *A* is incorrect because there is no indication of stress in Gulliver's tone. Choices *B* and *D* aren't the best answers because, though Gulliver seems fond of his new acquaintances, he didn't travel there with the intention of meeting new people or to express a definite love for them in this particular portion of the text.

21. C: The emperor made a definitive decision to expose Gulliver to their native customs. In this instance, the word *mind* was not related to a vote, question, or cognitive ability.

22. A: The assertion in Choice *A* does not support the fact that games are a commonplace event in this culture because it mentions conduct, not games. Choices *B*, *C*, and *D* are incorrect because these do support the fact that games are a commonplace event.

Writing

1. D. Choice *D* is correct because Sentence 7 incorrectly spells the possessive pronoun *their* as though it were the word *there*, which is not possessive. Since the sentence is describing the snow leopard's territory, the possessive pronoun *their* should be used.

2. B. Choice *B* is correct because Sentence 3 incorrectly uses the past tense phrase *was known*. Since the snow leopard is not extinct and the rest of the passage uses present tense, the sentence should use the present perfect tense: "However, the snow leopard has been known to make its home as far north as Mongolia and southern Russia."

3. A. Choice *A* is correct because Sentence 1 capitalizes *snow leopard*; however, it should not be capitalized because it is not a proper noun.

4. B. Choice *B* is correct because Sentence 2 has a spelling error in the plural noun *countries*.

5. C. Choice *C* is correct because Sentence 5 begins with the introductory dependent clause "Despite living on steep outcrops," which needs to be followed by a comma. The correct sentence should read, "Despite living on steep outcrops, the snow leopard is quite nimble and can cover a large distance in a short amount of time."

6. B. Choice *B* is correct because Sentence 6 incorrectly uses the adjective *much* in the phrase "as much as fifty square miles." The adjective *much* should only be used with singular, uncountable nouns. Since "fifty square miles" is plural and countable, the adjective *many* should be used: "Scientists have reported that female snow leopards can require as many as fifty square miles of habitat, with male snow leopards requiring as many as one hundred square miles."

7. D. Choice *D* is correct because Sentence 9 implies possession in the phrase "the snow leopards lifespan." An apostrophe should be added to the word *leopard's* to follow correct rules of possession.

8. C. Choice *C* is correct because Sentence 3 contains the clause "The coat is also incredibly thin," but the sentence goes on to say that the snow leopard's coat protects it from the cold. Using an adjective like *thick* instead of *thin* to describe the coat would improve the clarity of the sentence.

9. B. Choice *B* is correct because Sentence 4 contains the non-defining relative clause "which is nearly as long as its body" to describe the leopard's tail. As such, the clause should be enclosed with commas or em dashes: "Snow leopards also have a long tail—which is nearly as long as its body—and giant, padded paws."

10. B. Choice *B* is correct because Sentence 7 uses the adverb such as and has no verb, making it a dependent clause that cannot stand alone as a sentence. Combining Sentence 7 with the previous sentence will make a complete sentence: "For food, the snow leopard feasts on a variety of mountain-dwelling sheep and goats, such as bharal and mountain ibex, as well as small mammals and birds."

11. D. Choice *D* is correct because Sentence 5 describes how the snow leopard's features help it stalk its prey, and the additional sentence would provide more information about the snow leopard's hunting abilities. The new sentence would also fit with the one that would follow, Sentence 6, which describes specific types of prey. The sentences in the other choices describe different information, so adding the additional sentence after them would disrupt the passage's flow of information.

12. A. Choice *A* is correct because Sentence 1 contains the phrase "smokecolored coat." Since *smokecolored* is a union of two adjectives describing the noun *coat*, it should use a hyphen to form the compound adjective *smoke-colored*.

13. A. Choice *A* is correct because Sentence 5 contains the past tense verb *jumped*, which is not consistent with the present tense in the rest of the passage. The sentence could be corrected to use the continuous verb form *jumping* or the present tense phrase *it jumps*.

14. D. Choice *D* is correct because Sentence 9 uses verb tenses inconsistently in the clause "it will eat its fill and conserve its energy by lounging or to nap." The clause contains the continuous verb form *lounging*, followed by the infinitive verb form *to nap*. For consistency, the verb forms should be the same: "by lounging or napping."

15. D. Choice *D* is correct because Sentence 5 contains a spelling error in the word *commitment*.

16. A. Choice *A* is correct because Sentence 1 incorrectly uses the gerund *destroying*, which should be replaced with the noun *destruction*.

17. B. Choice *B* is correct because Sentence 3 refers to a specific year, which should be formatted as a numeral rather than spelled out: "As of the year 2022."

18. B. Choice *B* is correct because Sentence 2 includes a proper noun that is an institution name, so it should be capitalized in title case: "International Union for Conservation of Nature."

19. A. Choice *A* is correct because Sentence 4 uses the adjective *illegal* to describe the verb *hunting*. However, adverbs, not adjectives, should be used to describe verbs, so the sentence can be corrected by using the adverb *illegally*: "The snow leopard is legally classified as protected animal in many Asian countries and there are punishments like imprisonment and fines for illegally hunting and trading it."

20. D. Choice *D* is correct because Sentence 7 contains the clause "Zoos also continue fund breeding research," but the verb *fund* is functioning as an object of the sentence. Therefore, the infinitive form of the verb, *to fund*, should be used instead: "Zoos also continue to fund breeding research."

21. D. Choice *D* is correct because Sentence 6 is a run-on sentence consisting of two independent clauses that are jammed together without punctuation. Correctly punctuated, the sentence would contain two independent clauses joined by a coordinating conjunction: "[6]The use of non-invasive methods to study wild snow leopards is costly; however, scientists are committed to it."

Mathematics

1. C: The data points do not appear to form any sort of line, even approximately, as we would expect for a positive or negative relation. They also do not form the characteristic bell-shaped curve of a normal distribution. No relation is apparent.

2. D: The slope is given by the change in y divided by the change in x. Specifically, it's:

$$slope = \frac{y_2 - y_1}{x_2 - x_1}$$

The first point is $(-5, -3)$, and the second point is $(0, -1)$. Work from left to right when identifying coordinates. Thus, the point on the left is point 1 $(-5, -3)$ and the point on the right is point 2 $(0, -1)$.

Now we just need to plug those numbers into the equation:

$$slope = \frac{-1 - (-3)}{0 - (-5)}$$

It can be simplified to:

$$slope = \frac{-1 + 3}{0 + 5}$$

$$slope = \frac{2}{5}$$

3. B: The figure is composed of three sides of a square and a semicircle. The sides of the square are simply added:

$$8 \text{ in} + 8 \text{ in} + 8 \text{ in} = 24 \text{ in}$$

The circumference of a circle is found by the equation $C = 2\pi r$. The radius is 4 in, so the circumference of the circle is 25.13 in. Only half of the circle makes up the outer border of the figure (part of the perimeter), and half of 25.13 in is 12.565 in. Therefore, the total perimeter is:

$$24 \text{ in} + 12.565 \text{ in} = 36.565 \text{ in}$$

The other answer choices use the incorrect formula or fail to include all of the necessary sides.

4. A: The perimeter of a rectangle is $P = 2l + 2w$. We are told $P = 44$, so $2l + 2w = 44$. We are also told that the width is 2 cm less than the length: $w = l - 2$. Substituting this for w in the perimeter equation, we get $2l + 2(l - 2) = 44$, which is Choice *A*. Although it's not necessary to answer the test question, we could solve the equation to find the length and width. The equation simplifies to $4l - 4 = 44$, or $l = 12$, and since $w = l - 2$, we find $w = 10$.

5. B: To simplify the given equation, the first step is to make all exponents positive by moving them to the opposite place in the fraction. This expression becomes:

$$\frac{4b^3b^2}{a^1a^4} \times \frac{3a}{b}$$

Then the rules for exponents can be used to simplify. Multiplying the same bases means the exponents can be added. Dividing the same bases means the exponents are subtracted. Thus, after multiplying the exponents in the first fraction, the equation becomes:

$$\frac{4b^5}{a^5} \times \frac{3a}{b}$$

Therefore, we can first multiply to get:

$$\frac{12ab^5}{a^5b}$$

Then, simplifying yields:

$$12\frac{b^4}{a^4}$$

6. C: The product of two irrational numbers can be rational or irrational. Sometimes, the irrational parts of the two numbers cancel each other out, leaving a rational number. For example, $\sqrt{2} \times \sqrt{2} = 2$ because the roots cancel each other out. Technically, the product of two irrational numbers is a complex number, because real numbers are a type of complex number. However, Choice *D* is incorrect because the product of two irrational numbers is not an imaginary number.

7. B: The car is traveling at a speed of 5 meters per second. On the interval from 1 to 3 seconds, the position changes by 10 meters. This is 10 meters in 2 seconds, or 5 meters in each second.

8. C: The terms "whole numbers" and "natural numbers" include all the ordinary counting numbers (1, 2, 3, 4, 5, ...), and sometimes zero depending on the definition used, but no negative numbers. The term "integers" includes all those numbers, their negatives, and zero. So –4 is not a whole number or a natural number, but it is an integer. It is also rational because it can be written as a ratio of two integers $\left(-\frac{4}{1}\right)$; all integers are rational. It is a real number because it does not have an imaginary component (symbolized by the letter i); all integers are real numbers.

9. B:

$$4\frac{1}{3} + 3\frac{3}{4}$$

$$4 + 3 + \frac{1}{3} + \frac{3}{4}$$

$$7 + \frac{1}{3} + \frac{3}{4}$$

Adding the fractions gives:

$$\frac{1}{3} + \frac{3}{4}$$

$$\frac{4}{12} + \frac{9}{12}$$

$$\frac{13}{12} = 1 + \frac{1}{12}$$

Thus:

$$7 + \frac{1}{3} + \frac{3}{4} = 7 + 1 + \frac{1}{12}$$

$$8\frac{1}{12}$$

10. C: The average is calculated by adding all six numbers, then dividing by 6. The first five numbers have a sum of 25. This scenario can be expressed by the equation $\frac{(25+n)}{6} = 6$ where n is the unknown number. After multiplying both sides by 6, we get $25 + n = 36$, which means $n = 11$.

11. B: To convert miles to kilometers, we can multiply the number of miles by the miles-per-kilometer conversion factor:

$$4.67 \text{ mi} \times \frac{(1.609 \text{ km})}{(1 \text{ mi})} = 7.51403 \text{ km}$$

Because the question asks for an answer with three significant digits, 7.51 kilometers is the correct answer.

12. B: $\frac{5}{2} \div \frac{1}{3} = \frac{5}{2} \times \frac{3}{1} = \frac{15}{2} = 7.5$.

13. D: A given number divides evenly by each of its factors to produce an integer (no decimals). The numbers 5, 7, 8, 9, 10, and 11 do not divide evenly into 12. Therefore, these numbers are not factors.

14. A: The hundredths place value is located two digits to the right of the decimal point (the digit 9 in the original number). The digit to the right of the place value is examined to decide whether to round up or keep the digit. In this case, the digit 6 is greater than 5, so the hundredth place is rounded up. When rounding up, if the digit to be increased is a 9, the digit to its left is increased by one, and the digit in the desired place value is made a zero. Therefore, the number is rounded to 847.90.

15. B: Fractions must have like denominators to be added. The common denominator is the least common multiple (LCM) of the two original denominators. In this case, the LCM is 15, so both fractions should be changed to equivalent fractions with a denominator of 15. Multiply the bottom of each fraction by whatever number is needed to produce 15 and multiply the top of each fraction by that same number:

$$\frac{1 \times 5}{3 \times 5} = \frac{5}{15} \text{ and } \frac{2 \times 3}{5 \times 3} = \frac{6}{15}$$

Now, add the numerators and keep the denominator the same:

$$\frac{5}{15} + \frac{6}{15} = \frac{11}{15}$$

16. C: To find a common denominator, look for a number that has both denominators (12 and 9) as factors. 36 works. Multiply the top and bottom of each fraction by whatever number will make the denominator 36:

$$\frac{5}{12} \times \frac{3}{3} = \frac{15}{36} \text{ and } \frac{4}{9} \times \frac{4}{4} = \frac{16}{36}$$

Now that we have a common denominator, add the numerators.

$$\frac{15}{36} + \frac{16}{36} = \frac{15 + 16}{36} = \frac{31}{36}$$

Since 31 and 36 have no common factors except 1, this fraction can't be reduced.

17. A: Flip the second fraction and multiply.

$$\frac{4}{13} \times \frac{169}{27}$$

Simplify the fractions before multiplying to make the numbers simpler to work with.

$$\frac{4}{1} \times \frac{13}{27}$$

Multiply across the top and across the bottom.

$$\frac{4 \times 13}{1 \times 27} = \frac{52}{27}$$

The numerator and denominator do not have any factors in common, so this fraction cannot be reduced.

18. A: Divide 54 by 15:

$$\begin{array}{r} 3 \\ 15\overline{)54} \\ -45 \\ \hline 9 \end{array}$$

The result is 3 with a remainder of 9, which is equivalent to $3\frac{9}{15}$. Reduce the fraction $\frac{9}{15}$ for the final answer, $3\frac{3}{5}$.

19. A: Using the order of operations, multiplication and division are computed first from left to right. Multiplication is on the left; therefore, multiplication should be performed first.

20. D: The original number was 8 3/7. Multiply the denominator by the whole number portion. Add the numerator, and put the total over the original denominator.

$$\frac{(8 \times 7) + 3}{7} = \frac{59}{7}$$

21. B: The original number was $11\ \frac{5}{8}$. Multiply the denominator by the whole number portion. Add the numerator, and put the total over the original denominator.

$$\frac{(8 \times 11) + 5}{8} = \frac{93}{8}$$

22. B: To round 8.067 to the nearest tenth, use the digit in the hundredths place. The 6 in the hundredths place is greater than 5, so round up in the tenths place.

8.067

The 0 becomes a 1. Drop the digits after it.

8.1

23. A: We use the place value to the right of the thousandths place, which would be the ten-thousandths place. The value in the thousandths place is 7. The number in the place value to its right is greater than 4, so the 7 is bumped up to 8. Everything to its right is removed, which gives us 245.268.

24. C: It may help to look at this problem as a fraction: $\frac{1.2 \times 10^{12}}{3.0 \times 10^{8}}$. We can calculate $\frac{1.2}{3} = 0.4$, and using the rules of exponents, we can see that $\frac{10^{12}}{10^{8}} = 10^{12-8} = 10^{4}$. This gives us an answer of 0.4×10^4, which is Choice *A*, but our answer is not yet in scientific notation because the first term, 0.4, is not between 1 and 10. We can rewrite 0.4×10^4, multiplying the first term by 10 and subtracting 1 from the exponent, which gives 4.0×10^3, Choice *C*.

25. D: The slope from this equation is 50, and it is interpreted as the cost per gigabyte used. Since g represents the number of gigabytes and the equation is set equal to the cost in dollars, the slope relates these two values. For every gigabyte used on the phone, the bill goes up 50 dollars.

26. D: This problem can be solved by using unit conversions. The initial units are miles per minute. The final units need to be feet per second. Converting miles to feet uses the equivalence statement $1 \text{ mile} = 5{,}280 \text{ feet}$. Converting minutes to seconds uses the equivalence statement $1 \text{ minute} = 60 \text{ seconds}$. Setting up the ratios to convert the units is shown in the following equation:

$$\frac{72 \text{ miles}}{90 \text{ minutes}} \times \frac{1 \text{ minute}}{60 \text{ seconds}} \times \frac{5{,}280 \text{ feet}}{1 \text{ mile}} = 70.4 \text{ feet per second}$$

The initial units cancel out, and the new, desired units are left.

27. A: Convert these numbers to improper fractions: $\frac{11}{3} - \frac{9}{5}$. Take 15 as a common denominator:

$$\frac{11}{3} - \frac{9}{5} = \frac{55}{15} - \frac{27}{15} = \frac{28}{15} = 1\frac{13}{15}$$

28. A: Setting up a proportion is the easiest way to represent this situation. The proportion is $\frac{20}{x} = \frac{40}{100}$, and cross-multiplication can be used to solve for x. Here, $40x = 2{,}000$, so $x = 50$.

Science

1. A: The sensory threshold is the smallest amount of stimulus that is required for an individual to experience one of the senses. For example, during a hearing test, the sensory threshold would be the quietest sound that a person could detect. This threshold is an important indicator of whether a person's senses are working within a normal range.

2. C: Generally, all sensory pathways that extend from the sensory receptor to the brain are composed of three long neurons called the primary, secondary, and tertiary neurons. The primary one stretches from the sensory receptor to the dorsal root ganglion of the spinal nerve; the secondary one stretches from the cell body of the primary neuron to the spinal cord or the brain stem; the tertiary one stretches from the cell body of the secondary one into the thalamus. Each type of sense, such as touch, hearing, and vision, has a different pathway designed specifically for that sensation.

3. C: Visual processing begins in the retina. When an individual sees an image, it is taken in through the cornea and lens and then transmitted upside down onto the retina. The cells in the retina process what is being seen and then send signals to the ganglion cells, whose axons make up the optic nerve. The optic nerve cells connect the retina to the brain, which is where the processing of the visual information is completed and the images are returned to their proper orientation.

4. D: Veins carry oxygen-poor blood back to the heart. Intestines carry digested food through the body. Bronchioles are passageways that carry air from the nose and mouth to the lungs.

5. D: Catabolism is the process of breaking down large molecules into smaller molecules to release energy for work. Carbohydrates and fats are catabolized to provide energy for exercise and daily activities. Anabolism synthesizes larger molecules from smaller constituent building blocks. Bioenergetics and metabolism are more general terms involving overall energy production and usage.

6. A: All three types of muscle tissue (skeletal, cardiac, and smooth) share four important properties. They are contractile, meaning they can shorten and pull-on connective tissue; excitable, meaning they respond to stimuli; elastic, meaning they rebound to their original length after a contraction; and extensible, meaning they can be stretched repeatedly, but maintain the ability to contract. While skeletal muscle is under voluntary control, both cardiac and smooth muscle are involuntary.

7. D: The autonomic nervous system (ANS), a division of the peripheral nervous system (PNS), controls involuntary functions such as breathing, heart rate, blood pressure, digestion, and body temperature via the antagonistic parasympathetic and sympathetic nerves. Choices *A, B,* and *C* are incorrect because they describe characteristics of the somatic nervous system, which is the other division of the PNS. It controls skeletal muscles via afferent and efferent neurons. Afferent neurons carry sensory messages from skeletal muscles, skin, or sensory organs to the central nervous system (CNS), while efferent neurons relay motor messages from the central nervous system (CNS) to skeletal muscles, skin, or sensory organs. While skeletal muscle movement is under voluntary control, the somatic nervous system also plays a role in the involuntary reflex arc.

8. C: The sinuses function to warm, filter, and humidify air that is inhaled. Choice *A* is incorrect because mucus traps airborne pathogens. Choice *B* is incorrect because the epiglottis is the structure in the pharynx that covers the trachea during swallowing to prevent food from entering it. Lastly, Choice *D,* sweeping away pathogens and directing them toward the top of the trachea, is the function of cilia. Respiratory structures, such as the nasal passages and trachea, are lined with mucus and cilia.

9. B: The pelvic cavity is the area formed by the bones of the hip. Housed in that space are the urinary bladder, urethra, ureters, anus, and rectum. This hollow space also contains the uterus in females. The other body cavities listed contain other organs not specified in the question.

10. A: An alteration in the normal gene sequence is called a DNA point mutation. Mutations can be harmful, neutral, or even beneficial. Sometimes, as seen in natural selection, a genetic mutation can improve fitness, providing an adaptation that will aid in survival. DNA mutations can happen as a result of environmental damage, for example, from radiation or chemicals. Mutations can also happen during cell replication as a result of incorrect pairing of complementary nucleotides by DNA polymerase. There are also chromosomal mutations as well, where entire segments of chromosomes can be deleted, inverted, duplicated, or sent or received from a different chromosome.

11. B: According to the Punnett square, the child has a 2 out of 4, or 50%, chance of having A-type blood, since the dominant allele I^A is present in two of the four possible offspring. The type O blood allele is masked by the type A blood allele since it is recessive.

$I^A\,i$	ii
$I^A\,i$	ii

12. B: Dominant alleles are considered to have stronger phenotypes and, when mixed with recessive alleles, will mask the recessive trait. The recessive trait would only appear as the phenotype when the allele combination is aa because a dominant allele is not present to mask it.

13. B: The nephron is the structural and functional unit that creates and transports urine. The glomerulus, loop of Henle, and distal tubule are parts of the nephron involved in creating and transporting urine depending on their respective functions, so Choices *A*, *C*, and *D* are incorrect, as they represent only a part of the unit.

14. C: The uterus and ovaries aren't part of the birth canal, so Choices *A* and *D* are false. The cervix is the uppermost portion of the birth canal, so Choice *B* is incorrect, making Choice *C* the correct answer, as the vagina is the muscular tube on the lowermost portion of the birth canal that connects the exterior environment to the cervix.

15. D: Thyroid hormone is responsible for regulating metabolism, so Choice *D* is the correct answer. Insulin is involved in glucose uptake into tissues, testosterone is for sperm production and secondary male sexual characteristics, and adrenaline is responsible for mechanisms in the fight-or-flight response, making Choices *A, B*, and *C* incorrect.

16. C: The parathyroid gland impacts calcium levels by secreting parathyroid hormone (PTH). Osteoid gland is not a real gland. The pineal gland regulates sleep by secreting melatonin, and the thymus gland focuses on immunity. *Thyroid* would also be a correct answer choice as it influences the levels of circulating calcium.

17. D: Bone matrix is an intricate lattice of collagen fibers and mineral salts, particularly calcium and phosphorus. The mineral salts are strong but brittle, and the collagen fibers are weak but flexible, so the combination of the two makes bone resistant to shattering and able to withstand the normal forces applied to it.

18. C: The alveoli are small sac-shaped structures at the end of the bronchioles where gas exchange takes place. The bronchioles are tubes through which air travels. The kidneys and medulla oblongata do not directly affect oxygen and carbon dioxide exchange.

19. C: The pancreas functions as an exocrine gland because it secretes enzymes that break down food components. It also functions as an endocrine gland because it secretes hormones that regulate blood sugar levels. The kidney isn't a gland; it is an organ located directly below the adrenal glands. The stomach is an exocrine gland because it secretes hydrochloric acid. Like the kidney, the spleen is an organ, not a gland. Therefore, the only correct answer is *C*.

20. B: The endocrine system's organs are glands which are spread throughout the body. The endocrine system itself does not connect the organs or transport the hormones they secrete. Rather, the various glands secrete the hormone into the bloodstream and lets the cardiovascular system pump it throughout the body. The other three body systems each include a network throughout the body:

- Cardiovascular system: veins and arteries
- Immune system: lymphatic vessels (it also uses the circulatory system)
- Nervous system: nerve networks

Practice Tests #4 - #10

To keep the size of this book manageable, save paper, and provide a digital test-taking experience, the 4th -10th practice tests can be found online. Scan the QR code or go to this link to access it:

testprepbooks.com/online387/kaplan-nursing

SCAN ME

The first time you access the tests, you will need to register as a "new user" and verify your email address.

If you have any issues, please email support@testprepbooks.com.

Dear Kaplan Nursing Test Taker,

Thank you for purchasing this practice test book for your exam. We hope that we exceeded your expectations.

We strive to make our practice questions as similar as possible to what you will encounter on test day. With that being said, if you found something that you feel was not up to your standards, please send us an email and let us know.

We would also like to let you know about other books in our catalog that may interest you.

HESI

This can be found on Amazon: amazon.com/dp/1637751931

ATI TEAS 7

Amazon.com/dp/1637756402

CEN

amazon.com/dp/1637757891

We have study guides in a wide variety of fields. If the one you are looking for isn't listed above, then try searching for it on Amazon or send us an email.

Thanks Again and Happy Testing!
Product Development Team
support@testprepbooks.com

Online Resources

Included with your purchase are multiple online resources. This includes all seven practice tests in interactive format a convenient study timer to help you manage your time.

Scan the QR code or go to this link to access this content:

testprepbooks.com/online387/kaplan-nursing

SCAN ME

The first time you access the tests, you will need to register as a "new user" and verify your email address.

If you have any issues, please email support@testprepbooks.com.

Thank you for letting us be a part of your studying journey!

Made in the USA
Monee, IL
15 September 2026

63182436R00146